Health Behavior Change

Third Edition

Health Behavior Change
A Guide for Practitioners

Third Edition

Pip Mason BSc(Econ) MSocSc

Director of Pip Mason Consultancy Ltd, Birmingham, UK

Health Behavior Change, second edition, was placed Highly Commended in the category of Health and Social Care, British Medical Association Medical Book Awards, 2011

ELSEVIER

Edinburgh • London • New York • Oxford • Philadelphia • St Louis • Sydney • 2019

First edition 1999
Second edition 2010
Third edition 2019

Notices

Practitioners and researchers must always rely on their own experience and knowledge in evaluating and using any information, methods, compounds or experiments described herein. Because of rapid advances in the medical sciences, in particular, independent verification of diagnoses and drug dosages should be made. To the fullest extent of the law, no responsibility is assumed by Elsevier, authors, editors or contributors for any injury and/or damage to persons or property as a matter of products liability, negligence or otherwise, or from any use or operation of any methods, products, instructions, or ideas contained in the material herein.

Health Behavior Change, second edition, was placed Highly Commended in the category of Health and Social Care, British Medical Association Medical Book Awards, 2011

ISBN: 9780702077562

Printed in Great Britain
Last digit is the print number: 9   8   7   6   5   4   3   2

Content Strategist: Alison Taylor
Content Development Specialist: Kirsty Guest
Project Manager:
Design: Amy Buxton
Illustration Manager:

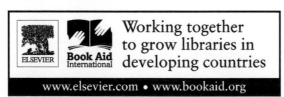

www.elsevier.com • www.bookaid.org

Contents

Biography

Pip Mason has a background in general nursing and her first post after qualifying was in neurosurgical intensive care. Quickly realizing that she was better suited to working with patients who were well enough to have a conversation, she took some counselling training and began working with people with alcohol problems.

From the start, she was intrigued by the issues of motivation, commitment, and ambivalence and enjoyed the challenge of engaging needy but reluctant service users. She was also intrigued by the emerging research showing the effectiveness of "brief interventions." These interests took her into work with other fields of addiction and into health behavior changes such as eating, physical activity, and medication compliance to prevent, and manage, both physical and mental ill-health. Her postgraduate research degree explored the value of placing alcohol counselors within primary care teams, something that was new at the time but is now widespread across the United Kingdom. She currently keeps her own consultation skills fresh working 2 days a week in a "recovery hub" in the West Midlands, UK, as a practitioner working with people who have gambling problems.

Her other developing interest was how best to train practitioners to work in line with the emerging evidence base. In a consultant capacity, she worked with the Health Education Authority (England) and World Health Organization, developing training packages and disseminating guidance on brief health promotion interventions to health professionals across Europe. Currently, she runs a training consultancy practice, Pip Mason Consultancy Ltd, teaching the ideas within this book alongside intervention skills such as cognitive behavioral therapy and motivational interviewing. For more than 20 years, she has been an active member of the Motivational Interviewing Network of Trainers (MINT), which is an international organization committed to promoting high-quality Motivational Interviewing practice and training. Many hundreds of people from all sorts of backgrounds have attended her courses over the years and shared their perspectives with her—some of their experiences arc found within this book.

Preface

The origin of this book goes back to the early 1990s when exciting and consistent research findings were emerging about the effectiveness of brief conversations between health professionals and their patients. It was becoming clear that notwithstanding the rigors of randomized controlled trials these mini doses of "talk therapy" could have significant effects on patient behavior such as drinking alcohol and smoking tobacco. Intriguingly the most difficult behavior change challenge was to get health professionals to integrate such conversations into their daily work once their research trial had come to an end.

It was at that time in Sydney, Australia, that I first met with Steve Rollnick. We were both overseas from our homes in the United Kingdom pursuing studies of various kinds into brief interventions, and we had several curious and meandering discussions on the topic. Putting ourselves in the health professionals' shoes we realized that the 5%−15% "success rates" of brief interventions, though impressive in public health terms, meant that approximately 90% of patients for a range of reasons did not fully follow their doctor's or nurses' advice. If they felt criticized or disrespected by the way the advice was given they might even change practitioners or put off future, needed attendances. Thus, the practitioners were not rewarded immediately or consistently for delivering brief interventions even though long-term results would be likely to reduce risk of harm to health.

This led us to wonder about what sometimes motivates health professionals to persist with unrewarding tasks and wondered if it was something about the nature of the transaction. For example, some nurses persisted for years in rubbing the backs of bedbound patients long after it had been shown to break down the already fragile skin. They did it because it felt immediately good both to give and receive a back rub. Their reward was a grateful patient and the warm glow of having done some nurturing. This appeared to outweigh their knowledge of how unhelpful it really was.

How could we use this insight? Both of us had backgrounds in counseling and person-centered therapeutic approaches and current interest in something called "motivational interviewing" which offered an approach to such tricky conversations in a psychotherapeutic setting. Could any of these or other ideas be used to inform the way short medical consultations were conducted? Could we make them feel inherently rewarding and congruent with everyone's wish for good relations between professionals and their patients? We already knew brief interventions worked if people did them. Was there a style of "doing them" that made them more likely to be done regularly?

We talked, wondered, looked out for other bits of the jigsaw that might help. We both returned home, and Steve drew a colleague Chris Butler into the continuing talking and wondering. As ideas began to emerge, we jokingly set ourselves the task of describing a conversation style that could be used in a 10-min time slot, be written on a page of A4 and taught in a lunchtime seminar. We did not quite make it. When you have read the book, you can judge for yourself how close we came!

We had a dream team: a primary care physician (Chris), a clinical psychologist (Steve), and a nurse (myself) each approaching the subject a little differently. We all had interests and responsibilities in terms of teaching at both undergraduate and postgraduate levels. We all firmly believed in the value of a patient-centered, respectful, and empowering approach to patients.

This is now the third edition and I hope we have, over the years, become clearer about our ideas and better at communicating them. The goal has been an easy-to-read handbook for busy practitioners bringing together a range of models and ideas, emphasizing common, useable threads rather than picking apart differences. We use ideas that can be used flexibly while still operating from a platform of evidence-based practice. Simple language has been used; we have not invented jargon terms or in any other way made it seem technical or esoteric. We know most people will dip in and out of a book like this and few will read it in the order intended. Consequently, we have occasionally repeated key content to ensure it gets read where needed to make sense of a chapter. Readers will of course skip over anything about which they do not need reminding!

Terminology is always a tricky topic in writing a book for a wide professional audience. The word "practitioner" has been used to encompass the whole range of health professionals, and the people they help are referred to as "patients." Spelling is an issue for books to be read on both sides of the Atlantic, and after discussion with the publishers, US spelling has been used. Apologies go to those who would have preferred us to make different decisions on these matters!

It was always a challenge for three of us to make time to collaborate on and jointly write a book. The first edition took many years. Since then Steve and Chris have had other demands on their time and energy resources, and I am left to develop this third edition of what will always be "OUR" book.

PM

Introduction

CHAPTER OUTLINE

Have you ever been frustrated trying to help a patient like Mrs. Burns?

Mrs. Burns has had heart problems in the past and gets very anxious when she gets breathless. Her doctor knows that her breathlessness now is mainly due to her inactivity. She rarely moves further than a trip to the kitchen to make a cup of tea (and she doesn't even do that if someone is there to do it for her). She sleeps and has a bathroom on the ground floor, so rarely climbs stairs. All of her caregivers have explained the value of gentle exercise to strengthen her heart and lungs, but she will not accept any suggestions to go for short walks around the park or shops, or to join a seniors' movement class. What her doctor sees as a behavioral problem, she sees as a medical problem that is out of her control.

Have you ever been delighted by a patient like Carlos Lopez?

Carlos developed back problems after an accident at work 5 years ago. Thorough investigations concluded that the best solution for him was exercise and pain management. Carlos was determined not to let his bad back rule his life, took all the advice given to him, built regular exercise into his daily routine and worked on cognitive strategies to manage his own response to the pain. He negotiated some changes in his job with his employers and is now back at work on a full-time basis, enjoying a full social and family life.

Have you ever felt discouraged trying to support someone like Sharon Barker?

Sharon wants to give up smoking. She is now on her fourth quit attempt. Her asthma nurse has offered all the support she can — referral to a support group, pharmaceuticals, nicotine replacement — but Sharon never lasts more than a few weeks before starting to sneak the odd one or two cigarettes, building to a complete relapse. She keeps trying and seems motivated, but nothing seems to work for her.

This book was written to make a difference in consultations with patients like these, based on an understanding of what works best. In recent decades, health practitioners have become more aware of how much patients can do to improve their own health, manage conditions such as asthma and diabetes and reduce the risk of compromising their health in the future. Increasingly, conversations in consulting rooms have focused less on what can be done to or for the patient and more on what patients can do for themselves.

Amongst the most frequently encountered *changes in behavior* which practitioners focus on are

- eat less, eat different things, adjust timing of meals
- drink less alcohol, abstain altogether
- be more physically active, do particular exercises
- smoke fewer cigarettes, abstain altogether
- take a new medication, a different one, replace one with another, at a different time
- monitor levels of glucose in the blood, ingest more/less liquid
- reduce intake of a drug, abstain altogether

Consultations about these changes occur in a wide range of *patients* who are, or who are thought to be

- at risk of suffering from heart disease
- recovering from a heart attack
- diabetic
- overweight or obese
- pregnant
- depressed
- at risk of contracting sexually transmitted diseases
- chronic pain sufferers
- people with irritable bowel syndrome
- problem drinkers

- substance misusers
- asthmatic

  The *practitioners* involved are usually

- doctors
- nurses
- nutritionists
- dietitians
- physiotherapists
- health visitors
- public health practitioners
- psychologists and psychiatrists
- counselors
- pharmacists
- fitness instructors
- dentists and dental hygienists

  The *settings* in which patients are seen are thus widespread and may include

- primary care
- inpatient
- outpatient
- community health projects
- emergency room
- leisure facilities
- occupational health clinics

BEHAVIOR CHANGE: THE HEART OF THE MATTER

Only patients can change their behavior, yet the practitioner can make things better or worse with every poorly or well-chosen word. This book is designed to help practitioners use every consultation well to increase the likelihood of a satisfying outcome and a healthier patient.

The logic with which the patient can be viewed as responsible for the outcome of a behavior change consultation has a formidable ring to it; after all, it is not the practitioners who need to change their behavior, is it? One can quite easily rationalize the process, thus: *What you* [the patient] *put in is what you get out*. This can take an aggressive form: *I can't help these people if they don't want to help themselves…*; or it can reflect a genuine desire not to impose one's values and will on the patient.

I'll help them if they want help, but if they don't, that's fine. … I respect the person more than I respect my right to tell them what to do (Primary care physician, aged 41).

Whatever our own approach to behavior change, we will continue to need to have such conversations with those we are trying to help. We cannot *control* the decisions our patients make, but we can talk and listen to them in ways that make matters better, or indeed worse.

PRACTITIONER MAKES MATTERS WORSE

Practitioner: Have you thought about losing some weight?

Patient: Yes, many times, but I can't seem to manage. It's my one comfort, my eggs in the morning, my fried chicken at lunch. I'm stuck in the house so much these days.

Practitioner: It would certainly help your blood pressure.

Patient: I know, but what do I do when I really want my usual big breakfast? It's a tradition in our family. [Sighs] I always get told to lose weight when I come to this clinic.

Practitioner: Have you thought about a gradual approach, like leaving out just one of the eggs for a while, and seeing what a difference it makes?

Patient: Yes, but how much difference will this make?

Practitioner: Over time, as you succeed with one thing, you can try another, and gradually your weight will come down.

Patient: Not in my house. The temptations are everywhere; you should just see what's on the table to munch, any time you want.

Practitioner: Have you talked to your partner about leaving these off the table, just to make it easier for you?

Patient: Yes, but…

PRACTITIONER MAKES MATTERS BETTER

Practitioner: Have you thought about losing some weight?

Patient: Yes, many times, but I can't seem to manage. It's my one comfort, my breakfast in the morning, my fried chicken at lunch. I'm stuck in the house so much these days.

Practitioner: It's not easy.

Patient: Say that again!

Practitioner: Some people prefer to change their eating, others to get more exercise. Both can help with losing weight. How do you really feel at the moment?

Patient: I'm not sure. I always get told to lose weight when I come to this clinic.

Practitioner: It's like we always know what's good for you, as if it's just a matter of going out there, and one, two, three, and you lose weight!

Patient: Exactly. I'm not sure I can change my eating right now. I used to get a lot more exercise, but life has changed and I've got lazy.

Practitioner: Well, I'm certainly not here to harangue you. In fact, all I want to do is understand how you really feel, and whether there is some way you can keep your blood pressure down. Perhaps there isn't at the moment?

Patient: Well, I could think about…

When patients fail to endorse practitioners' seemingly rational, friendly, and helpful advice, it is understandable that practitioners should feel frustrated or even blame the patients for irrational obstinacy. Indeed, a large body of research on compliance also appears to have embraced the notion that lack of success is basically a patient resistance problem (Butler et al., 1996). According to this model, the practitioner's role is to communicate information clearly, on the assumption that expert knowledge needs to be understood by the more or less passive and ignorant patients. However, the problem is not that simple, and patient resistance is not just a result of poor information delivery.

The imparting of expert knowledge is only one part of health promotion discussions. These days, in developed countries, people have good access to guidance on health behaviors and frequently know the basics of the practitioner's message, *eat well, drink less, move more, etc.* The practitioner moves quickly toward encouragement and being creative about making the task less onerous and more possible to maintain. How this is handled is critical to the outcome of the consultation. If resistance arises and the patient in the consultation does not seriously consider behavior change, the practitioner could well bear equal responsibility for this. If there is a specialist skill in the behavior change field, it is in the artful handling of this interchange, whatever the health behavior or pathology under discussion.

ORIGINS

The origins of this book go back to work in the field of brief intervention. Encouraging evidence began to emerge during the 1980s and 1990s about the effectiveness of routine brief advice from doctors and nurses to promote moderate drinking and smoking cessation. However, there was a twist; it seemed to be an uphill struggle, and many practitioners reported that implementation was tough and uncomfortable. One fear was that "nagging" sick people about their lifestyles might leave them feeling scolded and reluctant to return.

In searching for more constructive ways to build on this evidence, colleagues and I faced an embarrassment of riches. Despite awareness of time constraints in many settings and the complexity of many of the problems faced by practitioners, a framework came together with practical strategies that drew strength from a number of sources. Insights came from contact with practitioners in training, from being involved in research work, supported by the fields of patient-centered medicine and motivational interviewing.

The development of a patient-centered yet structured approach to medical care has been fundamental to our thinking about the rapport and relationship between patient and practitioner. See Constand et al. (2014) for a review of what is commonly meant by being "patient-centered." The website of the International Alliance of Patients' Organizations, www.iapo.org.uk, is a good source of information on this influential way of looking at health care. We have been interested to include wisdom from other related concepts. Concordance Dickinson et al. (1999) describes a shared understanding and agreement regarding the diagnosis, the therapeutic goals, and the choice of treatment. Achievement of concordance is helped by improved consultation skills. "Shared decision-making" also focuses on the collaborative processes at work, and Truglio-Londrigan et al. (2012) in their review paper state that "there is some evidence to suggest that shared decision-making does facilitate positive outcomes" and describe it as associated with "patient engagement, participation and partnership." It is not just doctors' interaction with patients that has been explored and discussed. Newell and Jordan (2015) review the evidence in relation to nurses in hospital medico-surgical wards and point to the "value and benefit of patient engagement…. The nurse-patient interaction is a core component of nursing science and high quality nursing care." Primary care medicine is expanding its scope. The practice of Social Prescription, reviewed by Bickerdike et al. (2017), takes a more holistic approach to lifestyle change signposting patients to local, nonclinical community resources that will support healthy behavior (e.g., contact with a befriending service to go on outings or giving free gym session vouchers, possibly to special sessions for those new to such work!). Solution-focused therapy, back in the 1970s, pioneered the idea of highly structured questions to influence the direction of the client's speech, and we are indebted to this approach for the scaling questions which we have adapted. Gingerich and Eisengrat (2000) give a review of the evidence for solution-focused work.

As the interest has grown in motivational interviewing, described by Miller and Rollnick (2012), it was of interest from the start to look at how some of the principles of this important approach could be integrated into a "good practice" structure for health professionals with a limited time frame in which to work and a narrower range of communication skills compared with the psychotherapy from which motivational interviewing was originally drawn. Over the years of exploring this style of consultation the evidence base for motivational interviewing in a medical setting has romped away. A couple of helpful meta-analyses are Vanbuskirk and Wetherall (2013) and Lundahl et al. (2013). Consequently, some key ideas have been integrated into the work here, and some of the ideas first published here in previous editions have been absorbed into motivational interviewing. Such symbiosis is probably inevitable and healthy.

This book does not claim to introduce lots of new concepts and ideas. The hope is that it draws on what we know of good practice and puts it all together in a manageable framework, a bridge between theory and research and the real-life challenges of clinical practice.

OVERVIEW

Fig. 1.1 shows an overview of the way in which we believe consultations can be structured. Each task is discussed in detail in the following chapters. Two obvious initial tasks are to *establish rapport* and to *set an agenda* (Chapter 3). The latter

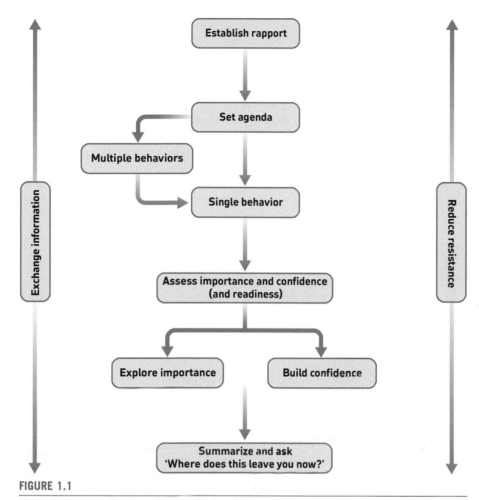

FIGURE 1.1

Key tasks in consultations about behavior change.

is sometimes unnecessary because practitioner and patient know what it is they wish to discuss. At other times, it is essential and often complex. The difference between single and multiple behavior consultations is here distinguished, the latter involving a delicate negotiation about the choice of topic: for example, smoking, eating, exercise, or some other personal concern.

Having agreed to discuss a particular change in behavior, the goal is to understand exactly how the patient feels about this. The task *assess importance and confidence* is designed to achieve this (Chapter 4). Some patients need more time to *explore the importance* of change (Mrs. Burns, mentioned earlier). Others are already convinced that they should change, and they want to, but need help to *build confidence* in their ability to achieve this (Sharon Barker, mentioned earlier). These are the next two tasks (Chapter 5). When they are completed, the next step will become clearer. It may be one of further exploration and discussion, or it may be planning the first step of an action plan.

There are two tasks which run right through the consultation process. These are *exchanging information* and *reducing resistance* (Chapter 6 and 7). Exchanging information will be used at various points to ensure that both practitioner and patient fully understand the key issues and each other's viewpoint. The patient might at any time show reluctance, defensiveness, or some other suggestion of resistance. This is an indication that all is not well in the consultation, and it might be necessary to change tack in some way, change the pace of the consultation or discuss this with the patient. All of these tasks are described in detail below, where we identify strategies that we have found useful to help the process along.

DOES THIS PARTICULAR APPROACH WORK?

We have drawn from a variety of sources, each of which has its own evidence base. This approach might be seen as a recipe, combining a variety of tried and tested ingredients. It seems that such a menu of strategies does improve outcome. For example, in the early days of developing brief interventions, Heather et al. (1996) found that a team of practitioners were able to make some headway with heavy drinkers on hospital wards, particularly those less ready to change. Butler et al. (1999) reported a similar good outcome amongst smokers in primary care. More recently, McCambridge and Strang (2004) produced strong evidence when a single, well-trained practitioner counseled at-risk college students, but progress was mixed when a group of youth workers had a single session with students (Gray et al., 2005). Other successful studies amongst young people have included work on diet (Berg-Smith et al., 1999) and children with diabetes (Channon et al., 2007). Tanner-Smith and Lipsey (2015) in a review and meta-analysis of brief alcohol interventions with young adults found that in the studies where specific strategies were used (including some described in this book), effects were larger.

Thus far, the evidence on the menu of strategies leads to a simple conclusion: skillful practice can make a difference to outcome, even amongst people who are normally quite difficult to reach.

One of the issues in doing such research is being able to define the intervention precisely and be sure that the study participants are delivering what you hope you are researching. Most reviews of the evidence end up commenting that in so many studies it is not possible to assess fidelity or to be clear exactly what the intervention really was. A helpful development was the Behaviour Change Counselling Index (BECCI) developed by Claire Lane (2002). It provides a single-page coding system to be used to measure the skills involved in behavior change counseling. It remains a useful document for both coaching/training and research. The manual and tool are available for free online.

HOW TO USE THIS BOOK
HOW MUCH TIME DO YOU HAVE?

This approach is designed to enable practitioners to learn behavior change consultation tasks to varying degrees of depth.

Just a few hours

Absorb the "spirit" of the approach (see Chapter 2) and familiarize yourself with some of the tasks identified in the single-page outline in Fig. 1.1. Identify the most useful tasks, and take note of some of the useful questions you might use in your consultations. These are listed in each chapter. Are you familiar with any of the typical clinical encounters described in Chapter 9? If so, these accounts will also give you a good idea of the overall spirit of the approach.

The website that accompanies this book (http://evolve.elsevier.com/Mason/healthbehavior/) has two video clips to watch. The first, "David" comes with a transcript and a commentary to help you follow the process. The second, "Ms Rees" comes with a worksheet posing questions for discussion in teams or private consideration. These questions are there to provoke discussion. "Right" answers are not given.

About a day

In addition to understanding the most suitable tasks, absorb some of the useful questions which are associated with each task. You should have time to explore some of the detailed strategies and visual aids associated with each task. Discussion with colleagues, preferably using simulated patients for practice, will help a lot. The website offers some tools to print off and use with patients to help structure the work.

More than a day

With this amount of time, you should be able to examine and practice the strategies embedded within the tasks. Practice these with simulated or real patients and return to the book for clarification and further reading.

WHAT SKILLS DO YOU HAVE ALREADY?

If you are reasonably familiar with the practice of using listening skills (e.g., open questions, summarizing, reflective listening), you should have no difficulty in learning to use the more directive strategies in this book. If not, it is strongly recommended that you work on developing your skill at listening first, as this is the fuel that drives a quality behavior change consultation. This is not saying, however, that you need to be an experienced counselor to succeed.

CREATIVE ADAPTATION, NOT SLAVISH ADOPTION

The collection of strategies in Chapters 3–8 are written out in a concrete form. The aim is to provide practitioners with a clear vision of what can work well. It certainly is not meant to imply that this is the only way, or always the best way, to proceed. Consider trying it this way first because it will help you get the feel of how to avoid reinforcing resistance and develop the discussion in a constructive way. When you feel more comfortable, adapt the strategy and make up new strategies that suit you and your patients. The context of your work might require considerable adaptation, in which case your collection will contain quite different strategies.

Some practitioners might want to integrate behavior change work into their everyday practice. Others might want to work on a particular project and develop a specific intervention: for example, for people with diabetes, obesity, heart disease, or nicotine dependence, or for improving adherence to medication more generally. The breadth of the approach described here demands pilot work, practice, and refinement. This should not be seen as a problem but as an opportunity to understand what is going on in your behavior change consultations. Seeking clarity, trying new ideas, becoming confused, and having discussions with others are activities that mirror what we would like patients to do. This is no coincidence because developing new ways of consulting involves changes in our own behavior. The evidence about practitioner behavior change points clearly to the need for piloting and practice, whether this be in the use of new guidelines or in developing patient-centered consulting methods. A method adapted and refined in-house by you will be more useful than one handed down to you from a book, a trainer or a manager.

REFERENCES

Berg-Smith, S.M., Stevens, V.J., Brown, K., et al., 1999. A brief motivational intervention to improve dietary adherence in adolescents. Health Education Research 14, 399–410.

Bickerdike, L., Booth, A., Wilson, P.M., Farley, K., Wright, K., April 7, 2017. Social prescribing: less rhetoric and more reality. A systematic review of the evidence. BMJ Open 7 (4).

Butler, C.C., Rollnick, S., Stott, N.C.H., 1996. The practitioner, the patient and resistance to change: recent ideas on compliance. Canadian Medical Association Journal 154, 1357–1362.

Butler, C., Rollnick, S., Cohen, D., Russell, I., Bachmann, M., Stott, N., 1999. Motivational consulting versus brief advice for smokers in general practice: a randomized trial. British Journal of General Practice 49, 611–616.

Channon, S., Huws-Thomas, M., Rollnick, S., et al., 2007. Multicenter randomized controlled trial of motivational interviewing in teenagers with diabetes. Diabetes Care 30, 1390–1395.

Constand, M.K., MacDermid, J.C., Dal Bello-Haas, V., Law, M., 2014. Scoping review of patient-centred care approaches in healthcare. BMC Health Services Research 14, 271.

Dickinson, D., Wilkie, P., Harris, M., September 18, 1999. Taking medicines: concordance is not compliance. BMJ 319 (7212), 787.

Gingerich, W., Eisengrat, S., 2000. Solution-focused brief therapy: a review of the outcome research. Family Process 39, 477–498.

Gray, E., McCambridge, J., Strang, J., 2005. The effectiveness of motivational interviewing delivered by youth workers in reducing drinking, cigarette and cannabis smoking among young people: quasi-experimental pilot study. Alcohol & Alcoholism 40, 535−539.

Heather, N., Rollnick, S., Bell, A., Richmond, R., 1996. Effects of brief counselling among heavy drinkers identified on general hospital wards. Drug and Alcohol Review 15, 29−38.

Lane, C., 2002. The Behaviour Change Counselling Index and Manual. University of Wales College of Medicine.

Lundahl, B., Moleni, T., Burke, B.L., Butters, R., Tollefson, D., Butler, C., Rollnick, S., November 2013. Motivational interviewing in medical care settings: a systematic review and meta analysis of randomized controlled trials. Patient Education and Counseling 931 (2), 157−168.

McCambridge, J., Strang, J., 2004. The efficacy of single-session motivational interviewing in reducing drug consumption and perceptions of drug-related risk and harm among young people: results from a multi-site cluster randomized trial. Addiction 99, 39−52.

Miller, W., Rollnick, S., 2012. Motivational Interviewing. Helping People Change. Guilford Press, New York.

Newell, S., Jordan, Z., January 2015. JBI Database System Reviews Implementation Reports 13 (1), 76−87.

Tanner-Smith, E.E., Lipsey, M.W., April 2015. Brief alcohol interventions for adolescents and young adults: a systematic review and meta-analysis. Journal of Substance Abuse Treatment 51, 1−18.

Truglio-Londrigan, M., Slyer, J.T., Singleton, J.K., Worral, P., 2012. JBI Library of Systematic Reviews 10 (58), 4633−4644.

Vanbuskirk, K.A., Wetherall, J.L., August 2014. Motivational interviewing with primary care populations; a systematic review and meta-analysis. Journal of Behavioral Medicine 37 (4), 768−780.

Principles

2

CHAPTER OUTLINE

INTRODUCTION

This book brings together the field of communication in health care, the study of motivation and how people change, and insights derived from listening to and observing patients and students. The book does not describe a new theoretical model or a specific protocol for consulting about behavior change. Rather, it offers suggestions on how to incorporate the fascinating things now known about this topic into everyday clinical practice.

It has been said, apparently since Ancient Greek times, that the three basic tools of medicine are "the herb," "the knife," and "the word" (Grant, 1995). This chapter is about the use of "the word" in behavior change consultations.

A lot has been written about good general consulting skills, much of which is clearly relevant to talking about behavior change. However, the behavior change consultation presents some unique challenges which make it quite different from, for example, the breaking of bad news to a patient or the eliciting of a history of presenting symptoms.

The aim of this chapter is to describe the principles on which the strategies described in the following chapters are based.

THE SPIRIT OF THIS APPROACH

A lot of attention is paid to technique and strategy in this book, yet by far the most important aspect is the spirit of the method. Put simply, this is a collaborative conversation about behavior change. Rather than wrestling, as a colleague once put it, it is more like dancing. The patient is encouraged to be an active decision-maker. The practitioner provides structure to the discussion (an "expert facilitator"), expert information where appropriate, and elicits from patients their views and aspirations about behavior change, helping them to become more aware of what is important to them and their intentions. This is not merely a matter of using techniques or strategies but of approaching the consultation and the topic of behavior change with a set of attitudes that promote patient autonomy.

Most of us behave, at times, in ways that compromise our health, and we each have our own notion of what constitutes acceptable risk. Most of the risks we take are for pleasure or some type of benefit, or we would not do it. Our clinical approach is based on the principle that, in general, people met by practitioners in consultations usually have the freedom of choice to behave as they wish, within the confines of their social and economic circumstances. Seen in this light, the role of the practitioner is to help patients to make an informed choice about whether or not to change their behavior. The practitioner might want to increase patients' knowledge of, and access to, healthy options, but their freedom to choose is their fundamental right. Most health-threatening behaviors are, after all, not illegal! If patients decide to change, it is the practitioner's role to help them to take effective action based on their choice. It is important to remember that most attempts to change behavior occur naturally, outside of the consultation. We all have experience of this in our own personal lives. Sometimes we succeed, and many times we fail. Many successful attempts only occur after a few "false starts." There is much to be learned from "failed" attempts to change that give people a better chance of changing in the future.

If your work is based on the principle that patients are to have as much autonomy as possible, it is not appropriate to force your views on them, however much you have their own best interests at heart. This approach is patient-centered but not without a clear structure and focus provided by the practitioner. Also, it does not mean that the practitioner should refrain from providing the patient with a clear, accessible account of the risks (and benefits) of health-threatening behavior. The practitioner's role is to help patients to make decisions that make sense within their own frame of reference. Your own views as a practitioner are nevertheless highly relevant. You do have knowledge about behavior change and about which behaviors are associated with optimal health. However, it is the way in which you share your knowledge with patients that is crucial. An appropriate approach to behavior change can be shown, thus: *What do you feel about your…? How does this fit into your everyday life? I believe that…, but it is your choice, whether to change or not. If you would like to consider change, remember, I am here to help you if you feel you need this.*

Sometimes, making decisions to change behavior can have profound effects on patients' lives. An idea like getting more exercise might seem simple to a practitioner but in fact can involve patients changing a lot in their lives. A practitioner was heard expressing frustration that his patients, overweight single mothers, would not take his "simple" advice to take a brisk half hour walk every day. He had not thought (or asked them) about the logistics of going out for even a leisurely walk with a baby in a stroller and a complaining toddler in tow.

Other behaviors might be affected, and the patient might need to examine fears about these changes; for example, *Will taking more exercise lead me to have a heart attack? Will giving up smoking make me put on weight?* Understanding these issues from the patient's point of view is crucial to the practitioner's efforts to promote change. To achieve this, it is necessary to keep close to a basic principle of patient-centered medicine; you must want to understand and value the patient's perspective. By seeing into the patient's world, process and outcomes will be improved. This is both a matter of attitude and technique.

It is crucial to respect the autonomy of patients and their freedom to change or to continue their behavior. Fundamental counseling skills can be used as a device for understanding, and demonstrating respect for, the patient's views. This is an active, not a passive, process, in which the practitioner tries to empathize with the patient or, in other words, to see the situation from their frame of reference. A patient may come from a different gender/cultural/social background from that of the practitioner and may have quite different, but equally valid, views and priorities. Conveying respect implies acceptance of whatever decision the patient takes about behavior change.

ASSUMPTIONS THAT CAN, IF WE ARE NOT CAREFUL, OBSTRUCT OUR WORK

Many behavior change consultations fail because the practitioner falls into the trap of making assumptions. Patients are more likely to consider change openly if you avoid imposing these assumptions on them.

This person OUGHT to change

This is difficult to avoid because you place a high value on health, you are concerned for the patient and their family, and often do feel that change would be a good idea. You cannot be dishonest about this but it may not be helpful to express it every time. The solution is either to hold back on giving your views until you understand those of the patient or to express them openly but not in an imposing manner: for example, *I think it is a good idea to change your diet, but what do you really think about this?* In other words, you can express your views in a relatively neutral and nonjudgmental way, placing emphasis on the patient's freedom of choice, while remaining open to the possibility that change, for them, may have negative consequences of which you are not yet aware. This also emphasizes that it is the patient's view that matters most. Having a fixed view that the patient ought to change can lead to a judgmental approach seeping through, the patient will then feel at a disadvantage and behave defensively.

This person WANTS to change

It is easy to assume that someone whose behavior is clearly making them ill, worsening a condition or putting them at risk will want to change. Turning up at a weight loss clinic or smoking cessation group is often taken to be evidence that people are well motivated to change. There are, of course, many reasons why people attend and many mixed motivations. The assessment of how much the person wants to change will be crucial to the success of the consultation. Remember that patients sometimes feel intimidated by health practitioners; they might not want to be frank because they fear possible disagreement about behavior change or fear being judged. The practitioner's general attitude and specific wording of questions can help to facilitate honest discussion. The risk of assuming that people want to change, without checking it out, is that of moving too fast into discussion of *how* they are going to change before they have really made a robust decision that they *want* to do so. Many are the times that practitioners are into action mode when patients are not yet at the point of deciding to change. Jumping ahead in this way can cause patients to feel misunderstood and badgered and increase their resistance to change.

Health is the prime motivating factor for patients

This is a very common faulty assumption made in consultations. We become entrapped by our own role as caregivers. For example, fairly healthy patients are not necessarily motivated to change behavior in the interests of long-term optimal health. More immediate prospects such as looking better, managing the household budget, or building a career might be more important. Changing behavior has implications beyond health, and not everyone is committed to avoiding poor health for as long as possible at all costs. You are also working in the context of uncertainties. You do not *know* that a particular overweight man *will* become diabetic or that his smoker wife *will* get lung cancer. You do know that their chances of doing so are greater and that behavior change would improve their odds of avoiding these diseases. They will make personal choices whether or not to take that gamble.

Approaches to risk-taking are fascinating. It is said that, in the United Kingdom, if you buy a ticket for the National Lottery in the last minute before they close the tills, your chance of winning the jackpot (about 14,000,000−1) is approximately the same as the chance of you dying before the draw, which takes place 2 h later. Millions of people buy tickets in the hope of winning, but no one has been heard to say it is not worth buying one, as they may not live to see the draw! When we tell patients that 50% of smokers will be killed prematurely by their smoking, some seriously consider those odds worth taking and reinforce this view by recalling all the smokers they know who were in the lucky 50% and died in old age from another cause. Assuming someone is motivated by health concerns can lead you to being blinkered regarding their real concerns and make it impossible to be patient-centered. Living for a shorter time but doing the things that really bring fulfillment could be what counts most for a lot of people.

If the patient does not decide to change, the consultation has failed

This assumption is unrealistic and overambitious. Deciding to change is a process, not an event, and it takes time. People vacillate between feeling ready to take action and feeling unwilling to even think about doing so. Simply helping someone to think a little more deeply about change is a useful outcome of a consultation. A decision to change is more likely to be taken later, outside of the consultation.

Management cultures based on targets put pressures on practitioners to get results. This pressure can get passed on to patients. In reality, it is not within your power to *make* people change. Thank goodness, the human spirit is too strong; ultimately, people follow their own lights, and even the most repressive and controlling regimes have dissidents. You may be right in considering you have failed if you omit to raise important issues with patients and do not give them a chance to think the matter through after taking account of relevant information. It is not within your power, however, to determine the outcome of that process. When you put pressure on yourself to get results, you can be so focused on the desired outcome that you do not pay enough attention to the interpersonal process and do not work as effectively as you might.

Patients are either motivated to change or not

Motivation to do something is not an all-or-nothing phenomenon; it is a matter of degree. Readiness to change varies between individuals and within them over time. In this approach, we have tried to incorporate ways to elicit any little sparks of interest in change from the patient, in the expectation that, over time, these might be fanned into flames. Someone who expresses little interest in change 1 day might be more interested a few weeks later. Similarly, the person who is really keen and committed 1 week may lose that enthusiasm later. Both scenarios are normal and to be expected. The issue of readiness to change is discussed in more detail below.

Now is the right time to consider change

Choosing the right time is a delicate matter and not always based on rational considerations. There is a common expression to "psych yourself up" for something. All sorts of practical and emotional factors affect people's willingness to consider change and feeling "psyched up" to do so. The best guideline is the patient's reactions. If he or she has rushed into the consulting room, late for work after a disagreement at home, you have a problem of timing. Practitioners are used to making quick decisions in their everyday work. It is not helpful to apply this approach (which is highly appropriate in dealing with acute medical problems) to discussion about a patient's change of lifestyle. Some change issues are urgent, such as HIV protective behaviors. A delay of a day or a week might really be dangerous. Others such as smoking might be, for some people, less urgent, although still very important. Choosing the right moment and moving ahead at the right pace will enhance success rates. Moving too fast can lead to patients digging their heels in. Also, working on change in an area other than that prioritized by the practitioner might be the best route to success for the patient. Smoking usually trumps most health-threatening behaviors in terms of adverse effects on health. However, if a patient is not ready to tackle smoking but is ready to consider eating more healthily, smoking could be "parked" for the meantime, and success in the area of eating could breed success later on in quitting smoking.

A tough approach is always best

How often have you been encouraged to change by someone who uses a tough approach? People take a hard line when they feel that no other approach is possible. With some patients, on some occasions, being very frank and directly persuasive might be justified and effective, but if we assume this to be necessary for every patient, our efforts will be wasted. Practitioners can enter a vicious circle when they use the tough approach; patients resist (because they do not like feeling cornered), the practitioner feels that they are inherently resistant to change, further tough action appears justified and so on. A *Yes, but…* response from the patient is almost a knee-jerk reaction to being told what to do.

I'm the expert. He or she must follow my advice

Of course you have expertise. You know what the literature says and have experience of what has worked for other patients in the past. You also understand the physiology of what is happening for the patient. It is not that practitioners' expertise is irrelevant, only that your role is to try to help patients to become more and more expert as well. Telling them what to do is unlikely to achieve this. Also, the way in which expertise is used is important. A useful analogy is that of a learner driver who employs a driving instructor. The pupil (or patient) does the driving, and the instructor watches, listens and encourages, making crucial decisions about where to go, how much information to provide and when to provide it. In consultations about behavior change, the patient should be in control. They need to practice and develop skills in being effective on their own. If we want people to take care of their own health in the long term, it is probably better to support them and offer information so that they can make their own decisions and plans.

The approach described in this book is always best

This is a generalization. A lot more clinical and scientific evidence is needed to justify such a statement. Some patients may respond to a much simpler approach, a kind but firm nudge in what you decide to be the right direction. The most successful practitioners are probably not those who stick slavishly to one way of working but who are flexible, skilled in different styles and sensitive enough to notice when they are doing something that is not helping the patient so that they can stop and do something different. This leads us on to discussion of the different consultation styles people use.

THE CONSULTING STYLE

A patient- or client-centered method has been constructed in many fields, for example, in psychology, nursing and medicine, where there is no shortage of evidence about the importance of taking into account the patient's perspective when making decisions about treatment and behavior change.

Among the most well-developed statements of the patient centered method is that provided by Stewart et al. (2003):

- Assessment is when the practitioner actively seeks to enter into the patient's world to understand his or her unique experiences of illness. The practitioner explores the patient's ideas about illness, how the patient feels about being ill, what he or she expects from the practitioner and how the illness affects the patient's functioning.
- Ideas about disease (abnormal pathology) and illness (the patient's experience of being unwell) are integrated with an understanding of the whole person in a broader context.
- Finding common ground involves both the patient and practitioner working together to define the problem, establish the goals of management and to be clear about the roles expected of the practitioner and the patient.
- Each contact between the practitioner and the patient is seen as an opportunity for health promotion.
- Each contact is an opportunity to develop a therapeutic relationship between the practitioner and the patient.
- Throughout, the practitioner is realistic about resources (including time and his or her own emotional energy).

Research support for the effectiveness of various elements of the patient-centered method includes demonstration of improved quality of the processes of care, increased patient satisfaction after seeing the practitioner, improved compliance with medication, reduction of patients' concerns, improved functional status, reduced use of tests, reduced use of emergency rooms and hospital admission, improved blood pressure control, improved postoperative recovery, reduction in blood sugar and improved well-being among people with diabetes (see Orth et al., 1987; Kaplan et al., 1989; Kinmonth et al., 1998; Stewart et al., 2000, 2003; Epstein et al., 2005, 2007; Hsiao and Boult, 2008). Interest has increased in the role organizations play in promoting a patient-centered approach and the importance of the health professional's skill and style. Ogden et al. (2017) studied "what organisational actions are required for patient-centred care to be achieved." However, our focus in this book is on individuals' communication skills.

THE STRENGTHS OF THE PATIENT

A subtle and powerful difference in your attitude starts to emerge as you encourage patients to harness their own ideas about behavior change; you find yourself working with their strengths rather than their weaknesses! You feel less like a problem- and pathology-seeker and more like a facilitator of their motivation to change.

One example of where this attitude is well expressed is in the delivery of the Nurse-Family Partnership project (see www.nursefamilypartnership.org). Here, an evidence-based program for young pregnant women is based on the fundamental principle that nurses work with the strengths and aspirations of the mothers; discussion of behavior change fits into what they want to achieve more broadly for themselves and their babies.

A more refined discussion of this topic can be found in the work of Dr Grant Corbett, who makes the distinction between "deficit" and "competence" worldviews. Within a deficit view, the patient is seen as missing things (knowledge, attitudes and skills) that the practitioner must rectify by filling in the gaps. Within the competence view, the patient is seen as someone with knowledge, attitudes and capabilities that the practitioner draws on as the primary focus for talk about behavior change (Corbett, 2006).

Patients sense your attitude toward them and respond accordingly. A genuine belief in their competence runs far deeper than being nice to them or even in trying to encourage them. It forms the very basis of the healing powers that you have to promote change, and it is infectious! Change will be more likely if you adopt a view of your patients as competent people facing tricky choices, via which they can make settled decisions.

FOLLOWING, DIRECTING, AND GUIDING

Rollnick et al. (2008) discuss three communication styles used in health-care consultations: following, directing and guiding. Each reflects a different way of looking at the relationship between a practitioner and a patient, and each offers the patient a different sort of help.

Following entails listening attentively to what the patient has to say about the issue to understand, as well as possible, their viewpoint. The patient leads the process and owns the agenda.

Directing is the process of telling people what they should do (with or without an explanation of why). When in a directing mode, we are working on the basis that we know best what should be done and how the patient should do it. The patient is expected to listen and comply.

Guiding is accompanying someone on their journey toward change and offering expert knowledge where appropriate. It is gentler than direction, and the patient has more autonomy. There has been a prior agreement regarding the agenda or destination, and the patient has consented to be guided in this direction.

All three styles are valid and useful in certain circumstances. Most health-care practitioners have skills in using all three styles and use a different balance depending on their role and preference. In hospice work and bereavement counseling, following might be a dominant style, as people are helped to come to terms with heartbreaking situations and find their own way through the dark times. In accident and emergency room work, a lot of appropriate directing might be heard as patients are told to *keep still, hold your arm out, swallow this*, while a crisis is managed. In health promotion consultations, guiding is probably the most useful style, as patients are helped to work out whether behavior change would feel worthwhile to them and how they could accommodate it in their lives.

A man who has had a heart attack is likely to be helped by each of these styles at different points, even within the same consultation. In the initial crisis when he is very frightened and does not know what to do to stay alive, he may be grateful for and comply with paramedics and emergency room staff's direction, trusting that they know best. Later, he may benefit from the following style of a nurse or hospital chaplain helping him talk through this brush with death and its meaning for him. Even later, a cardiac rehab dietitian might be able to help him, using a guiding style to work through the changes he might consider making to his diet.

Writers on concordance (Marinker and Shaw, 2003) have discussed similar ideas in the context of compliance with medication for long-term conditions. Traditionally, a role akin to directing has been taken by prescribers, and they have been repeatedly frustrated that patients do not take the medicines that evidence tells us would help. Concordance *refers to the creation of an agreement that respects the beliefs and wishes of the patient, and not to compliance − the following of instructions* (Marinker and Shaw, 2003).

The approach described in this book has most in common with guiding or concordance. It acknowledges the practitioner's expertise while deeply valuing the patient's input.

CHANGE IS A JOURNEY, NOT AN EVENT

There has been much interest over the last 35 years or so in exploring what leads up to someone making a change, and the factors affecting whether or not they maintain the change or revert back, eventually, to old habits.

The decision to stop smoking is, of course, always revocable. Once the smoker has embarked on an attempt to quit, he or she is repeatedly faced with another decision, namely whether to persevere with the attempt or abandon it (Sutton, 1989, p. 66).

For most patients, changing a health-related behavior is an ongoing process with which they need continuing support. A lot of thinking often goes on before they even make the first attempt to change, and maintaining change can remain a struggle for months or years.

In working on this approach, the literature on health psychology and behavior change was reviewed. Some themes stood out very clearly. First, the idea of *readiness*, derived from the stages of change model (Prochaska and DiClemente, 1983, 1986; DiClemente and Prochaska, 1998), was a useful starting point for understanding motivation and how best to work with patients. Depending on their degree of readiness to change, they have different needs, and it makes sense to respond accordingly.

Second, standing out from the different models of behavior change, many of them overlapping and in apparent conflict with one another, were two concepts, *importance* and *confidence*, which helped to explain a patient's degree of motivation or readiness to change. They appeared in different guises in different models but seemed to point to the same conclusion; if a change feels important to you, and you have the confidence to achieve it, you will feel more ready to have a go and be more likely to succeed. When sitting in front of patients, understanding their feelings about these three topics will lead to the heart of the complex forces that surround the topic of behavior change.

Readiness to change is a state of mind that reflects the outcome of quite a lot of psychological activity. For example, Joe keeps "forgetting" to renew his gym membership, Kim keeps his membership up-to-date and his gym bag in the back of the car but rarely finds time to go and Grenville makes excuses to leave work early so as to catch the late afternoon cardio class. They differ in their readiness to follow an exercise program.

Looking at how readiness varies in your work with patients is a useful starting point. Of course, you will want to know *why*, in the above examples and many others, differences in readiness arise. The concepts of importance and confidence should help with this task, and we will discuss these below. To begin with, however, we have been struck, like many other practitioners, by the value of simply being aware of this fluctuating and sometimes conflict-ridden state of mind, readiness. It has clear implications for how practitioners speak to people, whatever debate there might be about other aspects of the stages of change model (Davidson, 1998; Prochaska and DiClemente, 1998; Wilson and Schlam, 2004; West, 2006).

The transtheoretical stages of change model is an attempt to describe readiness and how people move toward making decisions and behavior change in their everyday lives. Its emergence in the field of health promotion and behavior change, which one commentator described as akin to the discovery of a new planet in astronomy (Stockwell, 1992), clearly struck a chord with practitioners and researchers alike. People, whether they are patients, practitioners, or the public at large, were described as moving through a series of stages when trying to change behavior, from precontemplation through to action and maintenance, along the lines illustrated in Fig. 2.1. A thorough attempt was also made to describe the process needed to move from one stage to the next, and the therapeutic techniques likely to engage these processes. Natalie Davies (2018) writes a concise overview and critique of the model and recent research on it in the context of substance misuse. For a full updated exploration of it from one of the original authors, see DiClemente (2018). The model is now so popular and well known; it may be unnecessary to spend time on it, but it can be worthwhile to revisit key concepts albeit briefly and acknowledge the large body of research backing its popularity.

If we take the example of smoking, which was used in developing this model, someone in the precontemplation stage can be expected to think and feel quite differently from someone in the preparation stage. While the former will not be

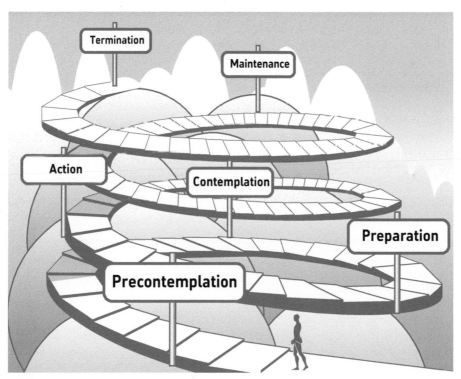

FIGURE 2.1

The stages of change model.

Adapted from Changing for Good by James O. Prochaska, John C. Norcross and Carlo C. DiClemente. © 1994 by James O. Prochaska, John C. Norcross and Carlo C. DiClemente. Reprinted by permission of HarperCollins Publishers.

actively thinking about stopping smoking, the latter will be planning very actively. Between these two people lies the person in the contemplation stage, who thinks about stopping, wants to do something about it but also does not. The model states that people are likely to move through these stages in the cyclical manner depicted in Fig. 2.1. The model, originally drawn as a circle, was later drawn as a spiral to demonstrate that, on relapse, people do not necessarily go "back to square one" but have the potential to learn from it and continue the journey onward and upward.

This model describes what happens to people as they change in everyday life with or without professional help. If we turn our attention to how one helps people who vary in their states of readiness, the usefulness of the model as a conceptual framework is striking; people have different needs and they do not all respond well to the same kind of help. Unfortunately, in the past, too many services have been action oriented, revolving around the small percentage of people who are ready to come forward and take action, typically less than 20% (DiClemente and Prochaska, 1998). The appeal of this model to practitioners probably does not lie in the precise definition of stages or the intricacies of stage-specific interventions but in the provision of general guidance; for example, if someone is not ready to change, action talk will be counterproductive. If this observation of the reason for its popularity is correct (see Rollnick, 1998), unresolved issues such as whether or not stages exist and how to match interventions to stages might not be critically important for the present purposes. Davies (2018) concludes her review, thus

Until something comes along to displace the cycle of change… perhaps it should be embraced for what it does rather than rejected for what it does-first and foremost, helping to understand and visualise the process, milestones and emotional labour involved {in change}.

The model provides a unifying concept, readiness to change, which is so clearly relevant to everyday practice that we should be able to use it as a platform for approaching behavior change.

In the context of substance misuse, that examination of the model helps researchers understand the larger processes of change where addict and treatment provider meet (DiClemente et al., 2004, p. 103).

In a more everyday context, a colleague described the model's usefulness as being similar to our understanding of the seasons. We cannot precisely determine when winter begins, and we can be surprised by a warm winter's day or a cold snap in summer, but the concept is still useful for deciding when to get the winter clothes out or get the garden furniture out of storage.

The challenge for practitioners is to maintain parity or congruence with the readiness to change of the individual. What happens when practitioners fail to achieve congruence, when they talk in a way that is not suited to the readiness of the patient? If we talk to a patient who is not thinking about change as if he or she is ready for action and keen to get as much help as possible, we will encounter resistance. Jumping ahead of the patient's readiness can be a risky activity. Resistance is discussed in more detail below.

For some years now, the stages of change framework has stimulated research and clinical development across a wide range of fields. Of particular interest are issues that revolve around the use of the stages of change model by practitioners to provide the rationale for intervention. The problem here is that making judgments about readiness, particularly if one is wedded to using stage labels, can be complex and have unfortunate, sometimes unintended, consequences. At best, these judgments are the outcome of genuine consensus between the practitioner and the patient. At worst, they can be oversimplified and driven by the prejudices of the practitioner. Four of the most commonly encountered difficulties are discussed below.

"LET'S NOT WASTE TIME ON THE PRECONTEMPLATORS"

Precontemplation, as noted above, is the first stage of change in the model developed by Prochaska and DiClemente (1983). We often hear the following sentiment expressed by practitioners: *If they are obviously not ready to change, leave them alone: concentrate your energies on those who are more ready to change.*

This interpretation of the stages of change model, as Ashworth (1997) has noted, can serve as a valuable stress reduction strategy.

... the model can provide a rationale for staff to give up struggling with those who are reluctant to change (Ashworth, 1997, p. 167).

In other words, one can avoid unnecessary conflict and reduce the workload by ignoring the precontemplators.

One can understand a busy practitioner, faced by a daily flood of faces, making this kind of decision on an individual basis about where to invest one's energy. Many a wise practitioner decides to leave an issue to one side in the hope of strengthening the relationship so that it can be tackled at a later date. However, it is one thing to make delicate decisions under time pressure, with the patient's interests firmly in mind; it is another altogether to adhere to a *general guideline*, which results in no discussion with precontemplators.

This practice is certainly not recommended in any of the writings of Prochaska, DiClemente and colleagues. In fact, they even talk of the need for a "paradigm" shift away from services which only focus on those who are ready to change (DiClemente and Prochaska, 1998). The main problem with neglecting to intervene with precontemplators is that you label patients with a stage-linked identity, almost like a trait, when you know their expressed feelings about change are context bound and changeable. You then descend into dichotomous thinking, for example, *people are either motivated or not*, and lose one of the most appealing features of the stages of change model, namely that practitioners need to be responsive to the wide range of patients' views and feelings about change. It then becomes fairly easy to justify not working with the "unmotivated."

This is what happened in the specialist addictions field for many decades; treatment was only geared around those who were really ready to change (a small minority). Patients expressing ambivalence were labeled as unmotivated and not amenable to help from an action-oriented treatment system. The possibility of finding ways of talking to less-ready sufferers remained buried beneath a sea of dogma (see Davies, 1979, 1981; Miller and Rollnick, 1991).

Patients labeled as precontemplators are quite diverse, an observation which led DiClemente (1991) to distinguish between reluctant, rebellious, resigned and rationalizing individuals. There might be ways of talking to such people without reinforcing resistance and disagreement. Indeed, a sensitive assessment of readiness, importance and confidence often facilitates achieving this goal. Interviews conducted among family practitioners who were trained to use this strategy reported positive experiences of its use, and this included talking about change among smokers who were far from ready to take action (Rollnick et al., 1997). Precontemplators might be more open to change than we think, a view supported by some of our research; heavy drinkers engaged in a health promotion discussion who were less ready to change fared better when faced with brief motivational interviewing than with a skills-based intervention (Heather et al., 1996). Along similar lines, we were surprised to find that smokers identified by practitioners as precontemplators responded better to an intervention based on the assessment of importance and confidence than to simple advice-giving (Butler et al., 1999).

DiClemente and Prochaska (1998) also report a number of studies in which it proved possible to improve retention rates among smoking precontemplators. To label people as precontemplators and decide that they are unlikely to benefit from an intervention could be unwise and premature.

READINESS TO DO WHAT?

Stage labels are frequently used by practitioners and researchers without clear reference to the exact nature of the behavior change in question. This gives rise to confusion and oversimplification.

Some behavior changes seem more complex than others. Stopping smoking is a relatively simple example, where a consultation often involves a single event, quitting. Making a judgment about readiness can be fairly straightforward. In contrast, with dietary changes, for example, there is usually not one but a range of changes to consider. These could involve adjustments, reductions, omissions, or new additions to eating behavior, or perhaps a combination of these strategies. Readiness to make these changes will vary. I might be very ready to eat more fruit, definitely not ready to eat less chocolate, and confused about the whole issue of reducing red meat intake. How will a practitioner judge my readiness to make dietary change?

The precise words you use are also important. Ask a heavy drinker how ready she feels about the following changes and you might emerge with different judgments about readiness: *How ready are you to talk about your drinking? … to think about changing your drinking habits? …to reduce your drinking on weekends? …to stop drinking once and for all?*

Many patients we talk to are considering changes not only in a specific behavior like eating, smoking, or drinking but also in other aspects of their lives as well. Readiness to change will vary across all of these potential changes, not just in the problem behavior. Ask the heavy drinker about her life as a whole, and you will emerge with different judgments about readiness. Thus, she might be a precontemplator in relation to complete abstinence (often the practitioner's main priority), a contemplator about reduced alcohol intake, in the preparation stage about eating healthier foods and in the action stage about ensuring that her children are better cared for.

Sometimes, particularly in chronic disease clinics, change or improvement is not a realistic goal for patients. Staying the same, or not getting worse, is what is talked about in consultations. A readiness assessment in these circumstances needs to be adjusted accordingly.

West (2006) is critical of the practice of using stage of change questionnaires to assess readiness and predict behavior. Agreed appreciating the usefulness of the stages of change concept does not equate to recommending the routine use of questionnaires in a consultation. Instead, a more conversational approach is suggested, using the model merely as a starting point for seeking congruence with the patient. Knowing which kind of question to ask requires skillful observation, judgment, a good sense of timing and careful listening. It seems clear, however, that judgments about readiness should be specific to a particular change. Beware the oversimplified use of judgments of readiness, particularly when an individual is assigned to a stage that hangs over him like a flag that determines how he is to be approached by a practitioner. For example, to label the above woman in trouble with alcohol as a precontemplator says only a little about her and quite a lot about the priorities and prejudices of the practitioner. We turn now to what is probably the most common example of this kind of thinking.

THE CONTEMPLATORS NEED "MOTIVATIONAL" HELP; THOSE MORE READY NEED A MORE PRACTICAL INTERVENTION

This focuses on how to match an intervention to the stage of change of the individual. In the past, practitioners and trainers, ourselves included, have presented this example of matching as one of the key messages of the stages of change model; contemplators need help to weigh the pros and cons of change (often called a *motivational intervention*), while those in the preparation stage need help with practical matters, such as techniques and strategies for improving confidence to cope with behavior change (*skills-based intervention*). Clinical guidelines have been based on this notion (e.g., Annis et al., 1996), and one major line of research into matching has investigated this hypothesis carefully (Heather et al., 1996; Project MATCH Research Group, 1997).

There seems to be some validity to this particular way of matching interventions to stages. Progression through stages does involve a shift in people's perceptions of the costs and benefits of change (Velicer et al., 1985; Prochaska, 1994; Prochaska et al., 2005), and less-ready smokers and heavy drinkers do seem to respond better to a less action-oriented discussion of change (Heather et al., 1996; Project MATCH Research Group, 1997; Butler et al., 1999). However, these research findings should not be overstated because the effects observed are not uniformly strong. Moreover, it has not emerged that those who are more ready to change respond better to a skills-based approach, despite the observation that self-efficacy is, according to Prochaska and DiClemente (1998), more important during the later stages of change.

There is a strong possibility that we have oversimplified the needs of people in different stages of change. Concerns about importance (pros and cons) are not necessarily restricted to the contemplation stage but can emerge in the preparation stage, an observation readily acknowledged by DiClemente and Prochaska (1998). Similarly, concern about confidence matters can also arise in the contemplation stage as we discovered in experimental consultations with smokers (Rollnick et al., 1997). Narrow stage-dose thinking, which restricts our attention in the contemplation stage to matters of importance (pros and cons), could undermine our work.

Linking motivational struggles to concerns about importance, whatever the person's stage of change, might also be ill advised. It implies that those concerned about confidence-building do not experience motivational problems. The term *motivation* itself, we suggest, should embrace both importance and confidence issues (see below) and be defined as equivalent to the more general concept of readiness to change.

WHITHER MATCHING?

The above discussion has centered on the idea of matching patients to treatments using the stages of change model. Can this notion be rescued from the kind of narrow stage-dose thinking described above?

Researchers have looked at matching interventions to stages quite carefully, a good example being the Project MATCH study which explored (among many other matching criteria) whether drinkers who are less ready to change do better with a form of motivational interviewing and, conversely, whether those who are more ready to change do better with a cognitive-behavioral approach or a Twelve Steps program. The results of this kind of study have been mixed (see Rollnick, 1998; Plotnikoff et al., 2007). An alternative pragmatic approach is to use generally tailored versus standardized interventions, in the hope of demonstrating that using the stages of change approach is better than a more conventional approach to intervention. Reviews of this work can be found in Ashworth (1997), DiClemente and Prochaska (1998) and Spencer et al. (2005, 2007). There is certainly something in this idea of matching according to readiness, but the findings could be stronger.

Could it be that these studies of matching are too far removed from what actually goes on in the consulting room and that the concept of matching is itself troublesome? Matching is not best achieved by giving a predefined dose of intervention to patients but by responding to changing needs on an ongoing basis in the consultation. In this sense, we could view matching simply as a process of maintaining congruence in the consultation (Rollnick, 1998). Sometimes, a contemplator likes to talk about the importance of change; at other times, about confidence. The same applies to people in the preparation stage. No wonder, then, that it has been difficult to locate matching effects in the studies by Heather et al. (1996) and the Project MATCH Research Group (1997).

In truth, this is about the delicate matter of how patients are spoken to and what specific changes they feel most ready to tackle. The best match is therefore not in some measurable characteristic of a patient, like readiness, or in some prepackaged intervention, but inside the consulting room, with the practitioner attempting to maintain congruence with the patients guiding them throughout their journey.

When we were developing this approach the stages of change model, with its call to pay attention to these matters, provoked thought about how to match the topic of conversation to the readiness to change of the patient. It was this challenge that led to experimentation with different topics in consultations and to review the literature on health psychology. These activities were stimulated by the question, *why* does a person place him- or herself at a particular point on the readiness continuum? There seems to be some common ground between the world of theory and clinical experience; people's feelings about whether change is worthwhile (importance) and whether they could achieve it (confidence) contribute to an understanding of readiness.

IMPORTANCE AND CONFIDENCE AS KEY ELEMENTS OF MOTIVATION

It has been helpful to make a distinction between importance (the *why* of change) and confidence (the *how* of change) for understanding a person's expressed readiness to change. This emerged not just from thinking about consultations but from a scrutiny of the literature where one encounters a bewildering range of overlapping theories; for example, reasoned action, self-efficacy, health beliefs, decisional balance and subjective expected utility theory, all of which looked at the question of why and how people change their behavior. It soon became clear that there is no single model that adequately explains the sometimes baffling complexity of behavior change (Butler et al., 1996). Neither is there one theory that is close to being uniformly endorsed by researchers and theorists. However, in self-efficacy theory, there was a useful framework that overlapped with many others.

Bandura (1977) developed a theory of behavior change based on two central concepts, efficacy and outcome expectations, but he then placed almost exclusive emphasis on the former during the next two decades. Efficacy expectations refer to a person's confidence in his or her ability to master a particular behavior change in a variety of circumstances, hence our decision to use the term *confidence*. This is not the same as a general concept like *self-confidence* or even *self-esteem*, which are more global concepts. *Self-efficacy* refers to a specific change and to a person's beliefs (whether or not they are well founded) about being able to cope with specific circumstances. *Outcome expectations*, on the other hand, refer to judgments about whether the change in question will lead to valued outcomes, hence our decision to use the term *importance*. In other words, someone is more likely to change a given behavior if he or she believes that, on balance, it will lead to good outcomes (importance) and also believes that across a range of situations, he or she will be able to master the skills needed to achieve that change (confidence).

References to the concept of outcome expectation abound in other models of behavior change. For example, reasoned action theory (Fishbein, 2008), the health belief model (Rosenstock et al., 1988) and the decisional balance model (Janis and Mann, 1977) have used different terms to describe a similar terrain: how people make judgments about the importance or value of behavior change. A more recent model embraces both the concept of self-efficacy and these outcome expectations of the value of change (see Schwarzer and Fuchs, 1995, 1996).

Having made a distinction between the *why* and *how* of change, there is nothing like a good dose of clinical reality to completely blur the distinction between them. Sometimes they do seem quite distinct, for example, when the perceived importance of change is markedly low while confidence is high. This is illustrated by a heavy drinker who anticipates no difficulty in reducing consumption (high confidence) but who does not feel that such a change would be worthwhile (low perceived importance). At other times, the two concepts interrelate, particularly when perceived importance is relatively high and confidence is low. Many smokers, for example, would very much like to quit but do not value the idea of change precisely because of the unpleasant perceived difficulties of coping with abstinence in difficult situations (i.e., low levels of perceived confidence). Quitting is not important enough to be worth the problems expected in its accomplishment. Moreover, as someone becomes increasingly ready to change, the *why* and *how* questions can collide, as reflected in the exasperation of someone who shrugs and says, *No, I just can't do it, it's not worth it*. However, clinical experience tells us that this does not render the distinction worthless.

In experimental consultations with smokers, they were asked why they placed themselves at a given point on a readiness continuum, and two themes emerged repeatedly, reflecting the issues of importance and confidence (Rollnick et al., 1997). In fact, there were even two smokers who placed themselves at around the same place on the continuum, who gave us very different answers to the question, *Why do you feel this way?* They both described themselves as midway along a readiness continuum: one, an elderly man who was very ill with a smoking-related disease said he was desperate to stop, it was very important to him, but he lacked the confidence to succeed; the other said that it was not very important to her to quit, but she had no doubt about her ability to succeed if she chose to quit smoking. Neither person was ready to stop, both being unsure about it all, but

BOX 2.1 THREE TOPICS IN TALK ABOUT BEHAVIOR CHANGE

Importance	Confidence	Readiness
Why?	How? What?	When?
Is it worthwhile?	Can I?	Should I do it now?
Why should I?	How will I do it?	What about other priorities?
How will I benefit?	How will I cope with X, Y and Z?	
What will change?		
At what cost?	Will I succeed if…?	
Do I really want to?	What change…?	
Will it make a difference?		

each for completely different reasons. We then found that the themes of readiness, importance and confidence echoed through conversations with people about changes in eating, exercise, drinking and even compulsive shopping.

Box 2.1 lists the kind of questions that people might ask themselves about readiness, importance and confidence. How to talk about these questions in a constructive way is our primary objective in this book. The terms *readiness*, *importance* and *confidence* are merely the keys that open the door to these discussions.

ARE THERE OTHER TERMS FOR THESE DIMENSIONS?

The decision to use the terms *importance* and *confidence* instead of the numerous alternatives available was driven partly by a desire to pursue simplicity of expression, to free practitioners from the weight of jargon that so bedevils some of the literature on behavior change. When it came to the term *importance*, we could have used alternatives like the *pros and cons* of change or the perceived *costs and benefits* of change. However, we wanted to avoid the potentially misleading impression that weighing up the value of change is a matter of balancing the rational components of something akin to a psychological ledger. It can be that simple sometimes, but this weighing up can also be influenced strongly by feelings about other matters beyond the behavior in question, often linked to fundamental values about health and well-being; hence our emphasis on the word *importance*. The term *confidence* instead of *ability* was used because it focuses on the person's underlying psychological state and avoids the mistake of assuming that talking about this topic is merely a matter of focusing on "technical" coping skills. So far, these seem to be the most useful terms. Practitioners working in languages other than English may need to experiment to find the most evocative translations.

COMPETING PRIORITIES

A person who is very overweight might feel that food is a comfort in the face of a difficult life in which well-being is undermined by a host of other problems.

The importance of a change in eating or exercise behavior is weighed up against the importance of change in other, sometimes more important, matters such as saving money by buying cheap food or being around and attentive to the children in the evenings, rather than going to a gym. This can be a difficult area to talk about, particularly if time is short. Other examples come from the world of chronic disease management. Many patients do not feel that they have a labeled condition like diabetes or asthma in the first place. This will obviously affect their feelings about the importance of changes in health behavior. Carers often find it nigh impossible to prioritize their own health over their caring responsibilities.

Under these circumstances, value conflict with the practitioner is not uncommon. A practitioner might feel that it is very important to look after one's health and prevent the onset of disease by adjusting one's lifestyle. Many patients, however, feel otherwise, for a range of reasons. These differences in values will influence beliefs about health and illness, attitudes toward scientific evidence and the perceived importance of a change in behavior.

THE RELATIONSHIP BETWEEN IMPORTANCE, CONFIDENCE, AND READINESS

Fig. 2.2 describes one way of viewing the links between these three terms, in which the patient's feelings about importance and confidence contribute to the more general state of readiness to change. These three concepts have a reasonably solid base in psychological theory. A review of behavior change research, in the addictions field and in health psychology, reveals a clear tendency for discussion to revolve around these concepts, particularly importance and confidence (see Chapter 5 for a fuller discussion).

In Fig. 2.3, if a group of people are excessive drinkers, they might all feel unready to change but for completely different reasons. Drinker A might feel that it is very important to change, perhaps because of a physical illness, but feel very

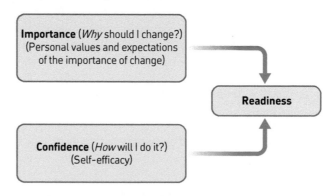

FIGURE 2.2

The ingredients of readiness to change.

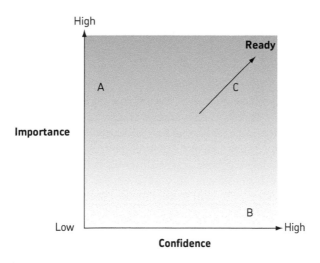

FIGURE 2.3

Readiness, importance and confidence: a practitioner's guide.

pessimistic about her ability to succeed. In contrast, Drinker B might feel confident that he could succeed with reduced consumption, were he to try, but does not feel it is important to do this at the present time. A third drinker, C, might have high levels of both importance and confidence and therefore be much more ready to change than Drinkers A and B.

The goal here is to provide practitioners with a conceptual aid for guiding conversations about change, not to construct a comprehensive model of behavior change. In the interests of science, it is tempting to make Fig. 2.3 much more complicated. Where, for example, are a wide range of contextual factors represented? In making decisions to change a specific behavior, patients have to take into account what will happen to their moods, other behaviors and other people. Everyday pressures, problems and pleasures do not disappear or remain static when we make changes in a particular behavior.

However, in the consulting room, the practitioner does not experience these contextual forces as separate from feelings about importance, confidence and readiness. In fact, conversations about importance, confidence and readiness usually form the channels through which contextual forces are expressed; they become the keys to unlocking the personal context in which the behavior occurs. For example, ask a patient about importance, and the conversation might focus on the specific behavior or it might turn to talk about personal values, other priorities, or the effect of change on something else like stress levels, a close relationship and so on. Talk about confidence to achieve change, and contextual matters will tumble down into the consulting room. Suddenly, for example, loneliness might emerge as a bigger priority than behavior change. Similarly, talk about readiness, particularly if the patient is close to decision-making, and the discussion will turn to matters of timing and other priorities. The value of these concepts lies precisely in the opportunity they provide to talk about the context in which the behavior in question occurs.

One clear limitation of Fig. 2.2 and the above discussion of it is that like most models of behavior change in health psychology, the focus is only on a single behavior. The subtle interrelationships between health behaviors, which are the daily currency of talk in the consulting room, are thus not taken into account. A change in one behavior often affects others. While attempting to capture these challenges in a practical way, with the use of an agenda-setting strategy for dealing with multiple behaviors in Chapter 3, there remains a theoretical leap to consider how readiness, importance and confidence change across different behaviors in different circumstances. Building a bridge between theory and everyday practice is an uncomfortable journey, in which theoreticians will justifiably be concerned about oversimplification, and practitioners will react against jargon and what they see as needless complexity.

The approach described in subsequent chapters is based on a framework in which monitoring readiness is viewed as an ongoing background task in the consultation, with the assessment of importance and confidence forming a platform for constructive talk about change.

MANAGING THE INTERNAL CONFLICT

In developing this approach, the starting point has been a belief that when considering a behavior change, it is normal to feel at least two ways about it. We are torn in two directions. For example,

- I want to do it and I don't want to do it *I want to be fitter but know that going to the gym will be difficult and pretty unpleasant.*
- I want to do X and I also want to do Y and it's not possible to do both *I want to lose weight in order to feel better about myself and I also want to eat fast food because I prefer it and I'm too busy to cook.*
- I don't want X but I don't want Y either *I don't want to get complications from my diabetes but I don't want the fuss of managing my blood sugars either.*

It was a challenge to incorporate a way of managing this into this approach to behavior change. Ideas have been borrowed from motivational interviewing, which in turn have their roots in person-centered approaches to counseling and psychotherapy. Here we use the word *resistance* to refer to the side of the conflict that says, *Stop pushing me, I don't want to change, it's not worth it, it's too hard, I'd be giving up too much that I enjoy.*

It is one side of the conflict and it is demanding a voice. This voice will get stronger if the patient feels it is not being heard or acknowledged. Thus, if the health practitioner keeps talking about the benefits of change, the patient will oppose the balance by talking about how, on the other hand, it would be hard or undesirable. However, if the health practitioner listens to and acknowledges the reluctance that is showing as resistance, this may create space for the other side of the conflict to speak. Consider the two examples below. The patient is pregnant and smokes.

Nurse A: Have you thought about how much good it would do your baby if you were to give up smoking? We know a lot now about how much smoking harms the unborn child.

Patient: Well I have tried to cut down but there was nothing wrong with my first baby. He's fit as a fiddle and I smoked right through that pregnancy.

Nurse A: Yes, you were lucky that time, but you want to give this baby the best possible chance don't you?

Patient: Well, of course I do but I've been a smoker for so long and it really helps me cope with the stress of balancing looking after Jamie with going to work and so on. I really don't think I could just quit. The stress of me giving up will be harmful to the baby inside my body; I just know that quitting will make my body a horrible place for my baby to be…

Nurse A takes the side of change. She promotes the benefits of quitting, and consequently the patient opposes the balance by explaining how hard she would find it (resistance). The stage is set for the nurse and the patient to argue about the feasibility of quitting and for the patient to dig her heels in asserting that it is too much to ask.

Nurse B handles it differently:

Nurse B: I wonder if chatting for a moment about giving up smoking would be OK, now you're expecting a baby?

Patient: I thought this was coming! Well I've tried to cut down but it isn't easy.

Nurse B: I know. A lot of people say that quitting smoking is one of the hardest things they have had to do. What's the hardest part for you?

Patient: Smoking is the way I get a break and calm down when I'm stressed. If I were going to quit, I'd have to find another way to relax. Quitting would also be tough for my baby because of all the stress inside my body.

Nurse B: Yes, you've got a lot on your plate at the moment.

Patient: I have, but I suppose other people get stressed and manage it without smoking. Is it true what they say that you have to quit completely; cutting down doesn't work?

Nurse B: That is what most people find. What is your experience?

Nurse B listens to and acknowledges the barriers to change and that frees the patient up to explore possibilities.

Change is more likely to occur if the patient talks positively about its importance and the possibilities of changing. At first sight, it is subtle, but contrasting the above scenarios makes it easy to see big differences in the engagement and reactions of the patient. You want to create an environment where they express both sides of the internal conflict, not just their resistance. You want them to hear themselves talking positively about change. This is more powerful than it is for them to listen to you doing so. Chapter 7 discusses this in more detail.

THE DIFFERENCE BETWEEN ADVICE AND INFORMATION

The approach described here is based on the belief that expertise is lodged in both the practitioner and the patient. When each of them shares what they know, good decisions can be made. The practitioner will have access to scientific information, knowledge of treatment options and experience of what has been found helpful by previous patients. Patients are expert in their own lives. Sharing information with patients is important and responsible, but telling them what we think they should do with it (advice) does not fit well with the spirit of this approach.

Here is an example of advice, again in the context of smoking:

Practitioner: (Recommending a particular course of action) You've done well to cut your smoking down to two a day but you need to get rid of those last cigarettes. The only way to do it is to become a complete nonsmoker, plain and simple.

Patient: (Contributes own view) Well I do enjoy those two at the end of the evening when I'm winding down, and I feel so much better since I cut down from a pack a day, I was thinking I might be OK going on as I am. My brother quit a year ago and he still has one occasionally.

Practitioner: (Disputes patient's view and goes back to arguing for quitting) No you mustn't think like that. Before you know it, a bit of extra stress, and you'll be back to square one and you'll have wasted all this hard work.

As an alternative, here is an example of information exchange:

Practitioner: (Elicits from the patient what he thinks about it) You've done really well to get down from 20 a day to just two. How do you feel about quitting altogether sometime soon?

Patient: (Contributes own view) Well I was thinking to stick with just two at night for a while. I feel so much better, and if I could just hang on to those two, it would be great.

Practitioner: (Giving information from her professional experience) Well some people do manage to be occasional smokers. I know a couple of people who've managed it. Most people though, in my experience, do OK for a few weeks and gradually it creeps up until they end up smoking full-time again. (Then elicits the patient's experience again) What have you found yourself?

Patient: (Contributes information from his personal experience) Well, thinking about it, the last couple of times I tried I was still having the odd cigarette as a treat and it only lasted a month or so before I hit a bad patch at work, lots and lots of deadlines and pressure, and was back to smoking. Maybe I'm one of the people it doesn't work for. It's a shame; I'd like to be able to...

It is not that that advice-giving should be discarded altogether. Advice-giving is appropriately entrenched in many aspects of health care. Our comments here refer only to consultations about health behavior change, where it is easy for nursing or medical students to absorb the familiar modus operandi and develop advice-giving as a consulting habit. There is evidence which shows that simple advice can effect behavior change, perhaps more so in the fields of smoking and excessive drinking than eating or exercise (see, e.g., Stead et al., 2008). The concern is that only a small proportion of recipients respond, that it renders patients passive in the consultation and that giving advice can lead to the threat of disagreement in talk about behavior change. Analysis of consultations reveals that requests from patients for advice are relatively rare (Heritage and Sefi, 1992; Silverman, 1997).

Silverman (1997) describes a number of ways in which HIV counselors avoid being too personal when giving advice, for fear of being met with outright rejection from the patient; they couch their advice as if it is information, something Silverman called the *Advice as Information Sequence*. They also use the word *if* so as to give the patient freedom to turn down the advice, and they make oblique references to other people when delivering advice; for example, *What we say in this clinic is…* Thus, skillful advice-giving is often delicately steered to avoid outright rejection by the patient.

This is discussed in detail in Chapter 6, where a three-step sequence (elicit—provide—elicit) for information exchange is described.

LISTENING AS A KEY SKILL

One way of viewing the consultation is to distinguish between microskills, which are used moment-to-moment, and broader strategies that the practitioner uses to guide the whole process; one moves along two trajectories at the same time. Listening skills are used at the level of microskill on an ongoing basis, to ensure that the practitioner understands the patient and is as active as possible. The strategies, like those described in this book, enable one to give the consultation focus and direction.

Being patient-centered involves more than "being nice and polite" to patients. It involves careful listening. This is not a passive process but an active and, at times, demanding process. In behavior change consultations, one might spend time listening carefully to the patient's feelings about readiness, importance and confidence to make a particular change, or one might attend to other, often fundamental, issues like what it feels like to have a particular disease, to come to the consultation, to have a personal problem and so on.

In using a patient-centered approach, practitioners have the following goals:

- To encourage patients to express concerns, fears and expectations
- To help them to be more active in the consultation
- To allow them to articulate what information they require
- To give them greater control of decision-making and therefore responsibility, particularly important when talking about changes in their behavior
- To reach decisions jointly and ensure that goals are feasible

To achieve this, the practitioner needs to encourage, to be curious, to ask open questions and to avoid making decisions without checking first with the patient.

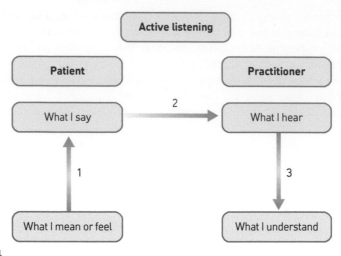

FIGURE 2.4

Active listening.

Much more subtle, and critical for the success of this kind of consultation, is the need to be a good active listener. Active listening involves searching for an understanding of the underlying meaning beneath the words used by the patient.

This process is illustrated in Fig. 2.4, which has been adapted from the work of Thomas Gordon (Gordon, 1970; Miller and Jackson, 1985). The aim is not to repeat what the patient has said, which is how a computer might carry out this task, but to clarify meaning, a more complex task.

Fig. 2.4 illustrates, from bottom left to bottom right, how the meaning being conveyed by the patient can get distorted: first, the patient might not say exactly what she means (see 1). At the second stage, the practitioner might not hear what is being said (see 2). Anyone familiar with strong argument will be familiar with this difficulty. *I said… No you didn't, you said…* Mishearing a single word can be sufficient to throw one off course. Third, one might hear the words accurately but interpret their meaning in quite a different way from the patient (see 3). Active listening involves bridging the gap between the two meaning boxes.

For example, if a patient says, *I find it comforting to eat the foods I like*, this could be taken to mean a wide range of things by the practitioner. To bridge the gap between the patient's meaning and the practitioner's interpretation involves careful listening and critically either making a statement designed to clarify meaning (sometimes called *reflective listening*), asking a question, or providing a short summary which clarifies the meaning.

Obviously, one needs to do much more than clarify meaning with patients. One might want to encourage exploration of options and decision-making, particularly relevant in talk about behavior change. There might be other things on the agenda of the practitioner. Consequently, the following chapters look at strategies for maintaining the focus and direction. This is a conversation with a purpose, and it is important not to lose sight of it. However, if the pursuit of patient concerns and meaning is left behind, communication breakdown will follow, usually in the form of resistance from the patient.

To listen well and to achieve the goals of a patient-centered approach, the following techniques are used:

- Simple open questions
- Listening and encouraging with verbal and nonverbal prompts
- Clarifying and summarizing
- Reflective statements, repeating, rephrasing, or paraphrasing what patients have said to encourage them to elaborate and to develop a better understanding of their meaning (see Rollnick et al., 2008 for further detail).

Examples of these skills are given throughout this book. Their acquisition requires practice and self-awareness of what one is doing and how the patient is responding. Some experienced practitioners say that practice taught them to make simpler contributions to a discussion, not more complex ones. For example, simple open questions like *What concerns do you have about your health?* or *What worries you most about this right now?* are usually more useful than complex questions like *How do you feel about the possibility of losing your good health in the future?* Experienced practitioners say that the less they follow their own agendas and hypotheses, the better they understand their patients. Simplicity of language is also more empowering for patients, particularly those with any cognitive impairment or neurological challenges.

For a detailed exploration of how the skill of listening can enhance our understanding of each other, see William R Miller's book on the topic (2018).

KEEPING FOCUSED

Having described the patient-centered approach, one might stop there and suggest that practitioners can now go forward into behavior change consultations armed with the essential tools of their trade, the patient-centered therapy of "the word." This might be inadequate for the following important reason: practitioners and patients often do not feel the same way about behavior change. There is often a tension, a potential for "disconcordance" that one can almost measure like the strength of an electrical current. A patient can resist pressure from a well-meaning practitioner to consider health behavior change. The different agendas of the practitioner and the patient can play themselves out in a conflict which is sometimes polite, sometimes hidden and repressed and sometimes open and hostile.

Behavior change consultations have a different quality from those that, for example, focus on breaking bad news to a patient. They are discussions about commitment and resolutions, strategies and obstacles, timing and fine-tuning and living one's life day by day, minute by minute for years to come. The subject of change is often raised by the practitioner, not by the patient, and resistance from the patient is thus much more likely. Moral judgments can be close to the surface of the discussion. Attention is usually focused on what the patient might *do* outside the consulting room. For these reasons, we feel that practitioners need structure to their consultations that provides them with a sense of direction, to help them avoid disagreement and achieve congruence with their patients. This is in the same way that car drivers, in addition to being able to start the car, steer it, change gear and apply the brakes, also need a map of some kind to ensure that they get to their destination. Good listening is an essential driving skill that helps the consultation to run smoothly. In addition to listening, practitioners need to guide the consultation in a helpful direction, to have some sort of map or structure to follow.

KEY POINTS

- Respect for autonomy of patients and their choices is paramount.
- The patient should decide what behavior, if any, to focus on.
- A confrontational interviewing style is generally unproductive.
- Information exchange is a critical skill.
- Readiness to change should be monitored continually.
- Importance and confidence should be assessed and responded to.
- *The practitioner* provides structure, direction and support; provides information wanted by the patient and elicits and respects the patient's views, negotiating change sensitively.
- *The patient* is an active decision-maker.

REFERENCES

Annis, H., Schober, R., Kelly, E., 1996. Matching addiction outpatient counseling to client readiness for change: the role of structured relapse prevention counseling. Experimental and Clinical Psychopharmacology 4, 37–45.

Ashworth, P., 1997. Breakthrough or bandwagon? Are interventions tailored to stage of change more effective than non-staged interventions? Health Education Journal 56, 166–174.

Bandura, A., 1977. Towards a unifying theory of behavior change. Psychological Review 84, 191–215.

Butler, C.C., Rollnick, S., Stott, N.C.H., 1996. The practitioner, the patient and resistance to change: recent ideas on compliance. Canadian Medical Association Journal 154, 1357–1362.

Butler, C.C., Rollnick, S., Cohen, D., Bachmann, M., Russell, I., Stott, N.C.H.S., 1999. Motivational consulting versus brief advice to quit smoking: a randomised trial. British Journal of General Practice 49, 611–616.

Corbett, G., 2006. What the research says about MI training: part II. Mint Bulletin 13, 14–16. www.motivationalinterview.org.

Davidson, R., 1998. The transtheoretical model: a critical overview. In: Miller, R.W., Heather, N. (Eds.), Treating Addictive Behaviors, second ed. Plenum, New York.

Davies, N., February 2018. A Step Too Far? Drink and Drug News, pp. 20–21.

Davies, P., 1979. Motivation, responsibility and sickness in the psychiatric treatment of alcoholism. British Journal of Psychiatry 134, 449–458.

Davies, P., 1981. Expectations and therapeutic practices in outpatient clinics for alcohol problems. British Journal of Addiction 76, 159—173.

DiClemente, C.C., 1991. Motivational interviewing and the stages of change. In: Miller, W.R., Rollnick, S. (Eds.), Motivational Interviewing. Guilford Press, New York.

DiClemente, C.C., Prochaska, J., 1998. Toward a comprehensive, transtheoretical model of change: stages of change and addictive behaviors. In: Miller, W.R., Heather, N. (Eds.), Treating Addictive Behaviors, second ed. Plenum, New York.

DiClemente, C.C., Schlundt, D., Gemmell, L., 2004. Readiness and stages of change in addiction treatment. American Journal on Addictions 13, 103—119.

DiClemente, C.C., 2018. Addiction and Change, second ed. The Guilford Press, New York.

Epstein, R.M., Franks, P., Shields, C.G., et al., 2005. Patient—centered communication and diagnostic testing. Annals of Family Medicine 3, 415—421.

Epstein, R.M., Shields, C.G., Franks, P., Meldrum, S.C., Feldman, M., Kravitz, R.L., 2007. Exploring and validating patient concerns: relation to prescribing for depression. Annals of Family Medicine 5, 21—28.

Fishbein, M., 2008. A reasoned action approach to health promotion. Medical Decision Making 28, 834—844.

Gordon, T., 1970. Parent Effectiveness Training. Wyden, New York.

Grant, V.J., 1995. Therapy of 'the word': new goals in teaching communication skills. Health Care Analysis 3, 71—74.

Heather, N., Rollnick, S., Bell, A., Richmond, R., 1996. Effects of brief counselling among male heavy drinkers identified on general hospital wards. Drug and Alcohol Review 15, 29—38.

Heritage, J., Sefi, S., 1992. Dilemmas of advice: aspects of the delivery and reception of advice in interactions between health visitors and first-time mothers. In: Drew, P., Heritage, J. (Eds.), Talk at Work: Interaction in Institutional Settings. Cambridge University Press, Cambridge.

Hsiao, C.J., Boult, C., 2008. Effects of quality on outcomes in primary care: a review of the literature. American Journal of Medical Quality 23, 302—310.

Janis, I.L., Mann, L., 1977. Decision Making: A Psychological Analysis of Conflict, Choice, and Commitment. Free Press, New York.

Kaplan, S.H., Greenfield, S., Ware, J.E., 1989. Assessing the effects of physician—patient interactions on the outcomes of chronic disease. Medical Care 27, S110—S127.

Kinmonth, A.L., Woodcock, A., Griffin, S., Spiegal, N., Campbell, M.J., 1998. Randomised controlled trial of patient centred care of diabetes in general practice: impact on current wellbeing and future disease risk. The Diabetes Care from Diagnosis Research Team. British Medical Journal 317, 1202—1208.

Marinker, M., Shaw, J., 2003. Not to be taken as directed. British Medical Journal 326, 348—349.

Miller, W.R., Jackson, K.A., 1985. Practical Psychology for Pastors: Toward More Effective Counseling. Prentice-Hall, Englewood Cliffs.

Miller, W.R., Rollnick, S., 1991. Motivational Interviewing: Preparing People to Change Addictive Behavior. Guilford Press, New York.

Miller, W.R., 2018. Listening Well, the Art of Empathic Understanding. Wipf and Stock, Eugene, Oregon.

Ogden, K., Barr, J., Greenfield, D., November 28, 2017. Determining requirements for patient-centred care: a participatory concept mapping study. BMC Health Service Res 17 (1), 780.

Orth, J.E., Stiles, W.B., Scherwitz, L., Hennrikus, D., Vallbona, C., 1987. Patient exposition and provider explanation in routine interviews and hypertensive patients' blood pressure control. Health Psychology 6, 29–42.

Plotnikoff, R.C., Brunet, S., Courneya, K.S., et al., 2007. The efficacy of stage-matched and standard public health materials for promoting physical activity in the workplace: the Physical Activity Workplace Study (Paws). American Journal of Health Promotion 21, 501–509.

Prochaska, J., DiClemente, C., 1983. Stages and processes of self-change of smoking: towards an integrated model of change. Journal of Consulting and Clinical Psychology 51, 390–395.

Prochaska, J.O., DiClemente, C.C., 1986. Towards a comprehensive model of change. In: Miller, W.R., Heather, N. (Eds.), Treating Addictive Behaviors: Processes of Change. Plenum, New York.

Prochaska, J.O., 1994. Strong and weak principles for progressing from precontemplation to action on the basis of twelve problem behaviours. Health Psychology 13, 47–51.

Prochaska, J., DiClemente, C., 1998. Comments, criteria and creating better models: in response to Davidson. In: Miller, W.R., Heather, N. (Eds.), Treating Addictive Behaviors, second ed. Plenum, New York.

Prochaska, J.M., Paiva, A.L., Padula, J.A., et al., 2005. Assessing emotional readiness for adoption using the transtheoretical model. Children and Youth Services Review 27, 135–152.

Project MATCH Research Group, 1997. Matching alcohol treatment to client heterogenity: project MATCH post treatment drinking outcomes. Journal of Studies on Alcohol 58, 7–29.

Rollnick, S., 1998. Readiness, importance and confidence: critical conditions of change in treatment. In: Miller, W.R., Heather, N. (Eds.), Treating Addictive Behaviors, second ed. Plenum, New York.

Rollnick, S., Butler, C.C., Stott, N., 1997. Helping smokers make decisions: the enhancement of brief intervention for general medical practice. Patient Education and Counseling 31, 191–203.

Rollnick, S., Miller, W.R., Butler, C.C., 2008. Motivational Interviewing in Health Care: Helping Patients Change Behavior. Guilford Press, New York.

Rosenstock, I.M., Strecher, V.J., Becker, M.H., 1988. Social learning theory and the health belief model. Health Education and Behavior 15, 175–183.

Schwarzer, R., Fuchs, R., 1995. Changing risk behaviors and adopting health behaviors: the role of self-efficacy beliefs. In: Bandura, A. (Ed.), Self-Efficacy in Changing Societies. Cambridge University Press, New York.

Schwarzer, R., Fuchs, R., 1996. Self-efficacy and health behaviours. In: Conner, M., Norman, P. (Eds.), Predicting Health Behaviour: Research and Practice with Social Cognition Models. Open University Press, Buckingham.

Silverman, D., 1997. Discourses in Counselling: HIV Counselling as Social Interaction. Sage, London.

Spencer, L., Pagell, F., Adams, T., 2005. Applying the transtheoretical model to cancer screening behavior. American Journal of Health Behavior 29, 36–56.

Spencer, L., Wharton, C., Moyle, S., Adams, T., 2007. The transtheoretical model as applied to dietary behaviour and outcomes. Nutrition Research Reviews 20, 46–73.

Stead, L.F., Bergson, G., Lancaster, T., 2008. Physician advice for smoking cessation. Cochrane Database of Systematic Reviews (2), CD000165.

Stewart, M., Brown, J.B., Donner, A., et al., 2000. The impact of patient-centered care on outcomes. Journal of Family Practice 49, 796–804.

Stewart, M., Belle Brown, J., Weston, W.W., McWhinney, I.R., 2003. Patient-Centered Medicine: Transforming the Clinical Method. Radcliffe, Oxford.

Stockwell, T., 1992. Models of change, heavenly bodies and weltanschuungs. British Journal of Addiction 87, 830–831.

Sutton, S., 1989. Relapse following smoking cessation. In: Gossop, M. (Ed.), Relapse and Addictive Behaviour. Routledge, London.

Velicer, W.F., DiClemente, C.C., Prochaska, J.O., Brandenburg, N., 1985. Decisional balance measure for assessing and predicting smoking status. Journal of Personality and Social Psychology 48, 1279–1289.

West, R., 2006. Theory of Addiction. Blackwell, Oxford.

Wilson, G.T., Schlam, T.R., 2004. The transtheoretical model and motivational interviewing in the treatment of eating and weight disorders. Clinical Psychology Review 24, 361–378.

FURTHER READING

Miller, W.R., Heather, N. (Eds.), 1998. Treating Addictive Behaviors, second ed. Plenum, New York.

Getting started: rapport and agendas

CHAPTER OUTLINE

INTRODUCTION

Practitioner: Your blood pressure is higher than it was last time.
Patient: Really? I feel OK.
Practitioner: Well it is definitely up. Are you taking the tablets regularly?
Patient: Pretty well.
Practitioner: What about cutting down on the alcohol?
Patient: [Starting to look a bit defensive!] Yes, I'm trying to.
Practitioner: Are you sticking to the diet we gave you?
Patient: Trying to.

Sometimes it is difficult to get started on a discussion about behavior change. Good rapport is essential for an honest discussion and for constructive understanding of patients' behavior and openness to change. Rapport is sometimes quickly established or reestablished, and the agenda is often obvious. In some settings, for example, in primary health care, there may already be an existing relationship between the practitioner and the patient, and this will provide a backdrop to the current consultation. In other settings, such as a first appointment with a dietitian, a relationship will need to be established quickly. Rapport is easy to understand and recognize, although sometimes it is taken for granted, and it can be difficult to repair once damaged (Fig. 3.1; Box 3.1).

Along with establishing a general rapport is the need to agree the topic for discussion. This may involve raising the issue with patients and also giving them a chance to raise issues with the practitioner. Where there are several possible topics for discussion and time is limited, a choice will need to be made. How this is done can affect how empowered the patient feels during the rest of the consultation.

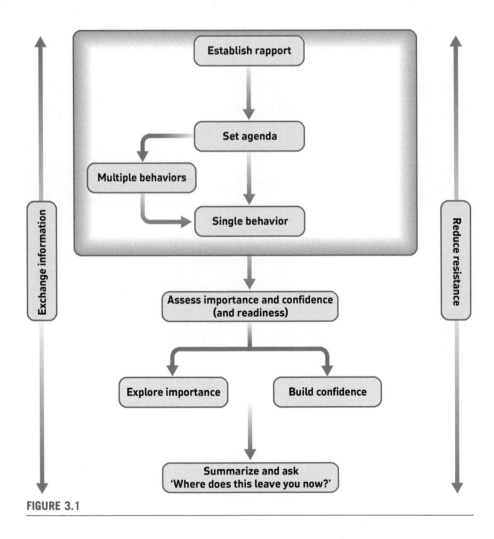

FIGURE 3.1

BOX 3.1 USEFUL QUESTIONS

1. What would you like to talk about today? We could talk about smoking, exercise, eating, or drinking, all of which affect your recovery from the heart attack. But what do you think? Perhaps you are more concerned about something else?
2. Would you like to talk about any changes to your health like eating or smoking, or have you come here today with other concerns on your mind?
3. Which of exercise or diet do you feel most ready to talk about?
4. Some people find that changing X [behavior] can improve Y [condition]. What do you think?
5. I am concerned about your chest. I wonder how you feel about your smoking?
6. How does your use of alcohol affect this problem [the presenting complaint]? What have you noticed?

WHAT TO AVOID

It is best to avoid launching straight into the topic before putting the patient at ease or establishing a climate of trust and collaboration.

Practitioner: [Looking at notes as patient enters] *So, have you given up smoking yet?*

ESTABLISHING RAPPORT

It is not difficult to get things off to a good start. Experienced health-care practitioners are often highly skilled at this. The guidelines below are basic but essential for avoiding damage to rapport. The most common cause for this damage is prematurely focusing on the topic that is of most interest to the practitioner, and this challenge will be discussed in the following section.

PHYSICAL SETTING

The physical setting for the consultation may either promote or obstruct development of a good rapport. An equal power relationship is essential if the consultation is to be conducted in the right spirit. Consider the following factors that may affect this:

- Is the patient's first encounter in the clinic one in which he or she will be listened to, even if just for a few minutes? Or are they obliged to undergo routine testing which is primarily of concern to the practitioner?
- Do they feel safe to talk? Is there appropriate privacy for patients (sound muffling as well as visual screening)? In some settings, such as pharmacist consultations at a drugstore, much physical work has been done to create environments conducive to health promotion work.
- Can the patient see the computer screen when entries are made in the notes?
- Do the wall posters create an appropriate ambience?
- Does the practitioner's style of dress unnecessarily suggest a power imbalance?

- Are patients unnecessarily in a vulnerable physical position that may lead to their feeling disempowered; for example, lying back in the dentist's chair wearing a bib?
- Has everyone in the room (e.g., students) been introduced?

THOUGHTS AND FEELINGS ABOUT THE CONSULTATION

Patients' expectations will affect rapport. They will expect or hope to be handled by the practitioner in a certain way. These can be checked and any misunderstandings clarified. Patients may also have come with immediate problems or concerns that will need addressing before they will be able to focus on other matters like behavior change. It is important to identify these and respond appropriately.

It is also worth acknowledging the context of the consultation for patients and their feelings about this: for example, *I'm sorry you've been kept waiting at the end of the day. I expect you're impatient to get home.* or *It must have been a worrying time for you since your heart attack [diabetes diagnosis, etc.] and I know you've already seen several other members of the team to discuss ways to keep you healthy in the future.*

It may be necessary to switch focus from treating the patient to guiding them to consider behavior change. After giving an injection, doing a dressing, scaling and polishing teeth, or some other procedure where the patient has (appropriately) been a more or less passive recipient of your ministrations, there will need to be a clear change in focus: *Now that's out of the way, let's sit down and think together about some of the other things affecting your...*

Some situations offer particular challenges. When someone has been very ill and has adjusted to being a compliant and passive patient, for example, after a heart attack, the move into a rehabilitation phase — *Let's look at what you can be doing to help yourself get better* — can feel like a real shift. In some health-care settings, patients have had a lot of their autonomy stripped away and have had to learn to be obedient. A secure psychiatric unit might be an example of this. Setting the scene for them to take some control over their health might be particularly challenging in such a context. If the patient feels respected and cared for from the beginning, any subsequent discussion will be easier.

ONE STRATEGY: A TYPICAL DAY

One useful strategy for establishing rapport is the *Typical Day* strategy, which is described in detail in Chapter 6 where its benefit to information exchange is highlighted. Here the patient describes a typical day and explains how the behavior under discussion fits into this context. The practitioner's role is to practice restraint and develop an interest in the layers of personal detail provided. It is also useful close to the beginning of a consultation, even if the subject of behavior change has not been raised. If one has time to spare, say 6—8 min, it can be a most worthwhile experience for both parties. One can follow the account of a typical day, in general, without reference to any behavior or can relate the account to a particular behavior: *Tell me what you might eat in a typical day.* If carried out skillfully, rapport will be strengthened immeasurably.

SETTING THE AGENDA

Jennifer, 35 years old and asthmatic, finds it very difficult to remember to take her medication regularly, smokes 20 cigarettes a day, lives in a family where all the adults smoke indoors and is very inactive. She says that after being on her feet all night, the last thing she wants to do in her spare time is exercise!

Sometimes there are so many things contributing to a person's poor health that it is difficult to know where to begin.

Of all the judgments made in a behavior change, the poorest often arise from a premature leap into specific discussion of a change when the patient is more concerned about something else. Indeed, this kind of premature leap can become almost institutionalized in a treatment setting, where patients are encouraged to change their behavior before they are ready to do so.

Sometimes it can be a relatively mundane matter that prevents a focus on behavior change; a patient who arrives at a consultation upset about a minor car accident might not be able to concentrate well on anything the practitioner says. Sometimes it is a personal matter that the patient is more concerned with and might want to talk about; someone who has recently had a heart attack might be preoccupied with matters of life and death. To talk about getting more exercise under these circumstances could be poorly timed, even insensitive. A critical early task therefore is to agree on the agenda.

Even when behavior change is a viable topic for discussion, one is often faced with multiple, interrelated health behaviors. For example, many excessive drinkers also smoke, and many who eat a fatty diet do little exercise. Thus, several health behaviors deemed to be risky often coexist in individuals. Sufferers from diabetes, heart disease, and other chronic conditions frequently face the challenge of more than one change. Deciding what to talk about first is thus a crucial initial step.

A distinction has been made in this chapter between single and multiple behavior change discussions when setting an agenda. It is suggested that practitioners make a clear and conscious choice between using either Strategy 1 (for multiple behaviors) or Strategy 2 (for a single behavior). This is because sometimes practitioners, when faced with a range of possible changes, prematurely oblige a patient to discuss one particular behavior at the expense of others. If someone is more ready to change their pattern of exercise than their diet, why focus on diet? At this stage of the consultation, the safest assumption is that the patient should be given control of its direction.

STRATEGY 1. MULTIPLE BEHAVIORS — AGENDA SETTING

Negotiating change is a specific process. It is applicable to a range of behaviors but can only be used with regard to one specific behavior at a time. It is not possible to effectively negotiate a "healthier lifestyle in general." We are all at different stages of readiness to change over different issues. Even within one topic such as diet, we may be ready to make one change (e.g., snack on fruit instead of chocolate) but not ready to make another (e.g., eat cereal or oatmeal/porridge for breakfast instead of bacon). Sometimes changing one behavior will have a positive effect on another, but it is important to keep the consultation process to one topic at a time. When there is a range of behaviors that could be discussed, it is essential to prioritize and focus on one clear objective. This makes the whole process more manageable. How do you decide what to talk about?

The guidelines for agenda setting with multiple behaviors are based on the use of an agenda-setting chart. This was originally developed in a general health promotion setting (Rollnick and Mason, 1992) and then refined and adapted by a team working on a negotiating method for use among sufferers from type 2 diabetes (see Stott et al., 1995).

WHAT TO AVOID

It is easy to be so focused on our own concerns that we do not notice that the patient has other priorities. When this happens, patients will either be disengaged or unenthusiastic about the behavior change consultation, waiting for an opportunity to raise their own issues. Alternatively, they will politely appear to comply with everything we say, without taking actually doing it because their own attention and concerns lie elsewhere.

The aim is to be open and honest about your agenda, to understand the patient's agenda, and to help the patient to select a behavior, if appropriate. The patient might, however, prefer to talk about a pressing personal matter. The practitioner's behavior and tone of voice should reflect an attitude of curiosity about what the patient really wants to talk about. This agenda setting can be done informally by asking a series of open questions. Here are some examples:

Before we get down to any details, what would you like to talk about? Changing your diet, getting more exercise, or maybe there is something else that's more pressing for you today?

What would you like to talk about today? We could talk about smoking, exercise, eating, or drinking, all of which affect your recovery from the heart attack. But what do you think? Perhaps you are more concerned about something else?

Can we just stand back a moment? Tell me how you would like to spend this time together. I usually talk to people in a situation like yours about smoking, food, exercise, medications and that sort of thing. How do you feel? Which of these do you feel most ready to change, or is there something else bothering you?

We have found that the use of an *agenda-setting chart* (Fig. 3.2) is one way of doing this. It not only saves time but also involves you in a collaborative exercise

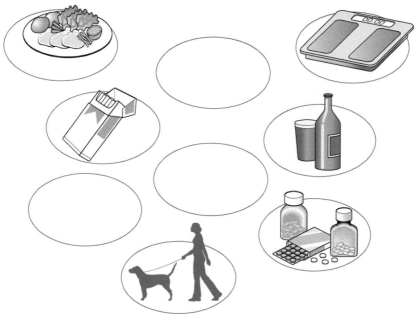

FIGURE 3.2

An agenda-setting chart.

Adapted from Stott, N.C.H., Rollnick, S., Rees, M., Pill, R., 1995. Innovation in clinical method: diabetes care and negotiating skills. Family Practice 12, 413–416, Fig. 1, Oxford University Press, with permission of the publisher.

that maximizes patient choice. Remember that this chart is merely an aid to dialog. The visual aid should not get in the way. It can be just as useful to conduct this negotiation without the chart by simply asking a set of open questions.

The agenda-setting chart illustrates a range of health behaviors. The chart has blank spaces on it to represent issues or behaviors which the patient feels might affect the possibility of behavior change; for example, a spouse who also smokes, financial worries which affect the purchase of different food, or a more pressing personal problem such as feeling depressed. Using the chart allows the practitioner to openly acknowledge what behaviors he or she is concerned about. The aim is to encourage the patient to decide what to talk about, assisted by the practitioner.

- You can draw a chart as you go, filling in the bubbles with topics raised by the patient or yourself. Alternatively, a preprepared card can be used. You can download this tool from the website (http://evolve.elsevier.com/Mason/healthbehavior/) or it can be photocopied from Appendices 1 and 2.
- It can be helpful to write on the chart or even to ask the patient to do so. For example, in the blank spaces, you can fill in a concern raised by the patient. You might cross out a behavior that is not relevant (e.g., *I've never smoked*) or check off something that they are already addressing (e.g., *I've already joined the gym and*

go every other day). Or you might even write a specific target underneath a circle and suggest that the patient take the chart home. On the website (http://evolve. elsevier.com/Mason/healthbehavior/), you can watch this tool being used in this way with a patient, and the transcript of this consultation is given in Chapter 12.

- Exchanging information can be a crucial part of this review (see Chapter 6).
- The two most common dangers when using this chart are a tendency to use it as a checklist to be worked through painstakingly and being in a hurry, which usually leads to a premature focus on one behavior at the expense of others.
- The chart should not be given to practitioners without prior explanation of its purpose and use.

INTRODUCE THE AGENDA-SETTING CHART

Example: On this card is a range of things that can affect people's health. Those that most affect [patient's condition, if appropriate] are... How do you feel about these? Are you ready to think about changing any of them? These blank spaces are for any other issues that you think might be of greater concern to you today. What do you think? What would you like to talk about today?

Note that there is a difference between saying to the patient, *Are you ready to think about changing any of…?* (used above), and saying, *Are you ready to change any of…?* More patients will be responsive to the former approach than the latter, which demands a greater degree of readiness to change. Another example is as follows:

On this card here are some of the things that affect people's health. I wonder whether you might be interested in talking about changing your diet or smoking, but what do you think? You will be the best judge of what to consider changing. Are there any that you think we could talk about? Or do you have other concerns today [pointing to blank circles] that are more pressing? Where do you think is the best place to start?

Note the difference between *Where is the best place to start?* and *Which is the most important?*. Asking about the best place to start often identifies the one that feels most manageable, whereas the most important may well be the most impossible from the patient's perspective.

Practitioners sometimes feel anxious about letting the patient decide where to start. For example, it can be difficult to be talking about food to someone of normal weight who is smoking 30 cigarettes a day but does not want to consider quitting. This person might be willing to explore the possibility of eating healthier with a view to losing a few pounds, but this seems less of a priority to the practitioner. This raises interesting questions:

- Why do we think we know what would most improve someone else's quality of life?
- Realistically, can we insist on them prioritizing one behavior over another?

- If they have some success in changing one behavior, can we expect that to have a positive influence on their willingness, later, to change another?
- What about our duty of care when we think there are clear priorities?

What would we say to one of the world's most famous classical guitarists who once offered these reflections about his life?

I probably eat, drink and smoke more than I should, but then I enjoy life immensely which probably evens things out… nicotine slightly raises blood pressure, stimulating the red corpuscles under the fingernails, encouraging them to grow. On occasions when I have briefly stopped smoking, the tone of my playing has lost its bloom, because the nails are considerably weakened (The Guardian, 14 January 1997).

The approach in this book is based on the assumption that patients are usually the best judge of whether behavior change will be beneficial in terms of their own priorities.

Many practitioners handle such a situation by giving a clear message about their own perspective: *We do know that stopping smoking is the single most important thing you can do to improve your health and I do recommend that you think seriously about it*, but then returning responsibility to the patient: *But it is up to you to do what you think is best and the most manageable for you.*

DEAL WITH OTHER CONCERNS

Practitioners often say that the blank circles are the most useful part of the agenda-setting chart. If patients identify some other issue or concern, be careful not to assume that they want to talk about it at this time.

However, if the patient does want to talk about something, the challenge is to listen, give information and then decide where to go next, all in a brief period of time. Do not assume that because patients want to talk about an issue, they want a psychotherapy session! Patients are usually aware of time constraints, and a few minutes of careful listening is much appreciated. At a certain point, you, and hopefully the patient as well, will be happy to "park" this discussion. At that point, you might say something like *We have talked about…, and I can understand why this must be bothering you. Where does this leave us now? Would you be happy to move on to talk about other things?* It can be useful to write this concern into one of the blank spaces on the agenda-setting chart. This clearly acknowledges its importance and makes it easier for the patient to put it aside for now.

DISCUSS THE RANGE OF BEHAVIORS

Take care not to push the patient into a premature focus on any single behavior. Listen and elicit. Get yourself into a curious state of mind. You really want to know exactly how the person feels about the selection of a topic to talk about.

You can use the *readiness rule* (see p. 65, or it can be downloaded from the website (http://evolve.elsevier.com/Mason/healthbehavior/) or photocopied from Appendix 3) to help with this task. Your goal is to find out which behavior the patient is most ready to talk about. For example:

Which of these do you feel most ready to think about changing?

What exactly are you saying about your smoking and drinking? How ready do you feel to talk about changing them, or would you prefer to leave it for the time being?

Thinking about getting more exercise, where would you place yourself on this line? Some people are not at all ready, some are very ready, and others are somewhere in between. How do you feel about this at the moment?

SUMMARIZE THE OUTCOME

Summarize your understanding of the outcome, and be prepared for any of these possibilities:

- The patient is not interested in changing any behavior, in which case your discussion could end here.
- The patient is willing to talk about changing a specific behavior.
- The patient is ambivalent about a particular behavior.

Consider a more detailed examination of the importance of change and the building of confidence (Chapter 5). If time is running out, you might consider asking the patient to keep a diary of the behavior or simply to go away and think about it.

Practitioners can misunderstand the emphasis on patient autonomy and readiness to change in this stage of the consultation and indeed in all of the strategies described in this book. It can be used as a vehicle for reinforcing pessimism and even a form of passive aggression, borne of frustration from dealing with particularly difficult behavior change encounters: *It's not up to me; it's up to the patient. If he wants to die young, that's his problem.* We have encountered practitioners using the agenda-setting strategy described below with this kind of attitude toward the process. Besides the obvious need to take stock of one's own feelings about the lack of patient progress in one's work, it can be useful to remember that we are not talking here about being guided by a simple notion of directiveness versus nondirectiveness. The practitioner is very directive in using the agenda-setting strategy described above, in defining the task and seeing it through to a satisfactory outcome. At the same time, it is also a patient-centered tool, as it encourages the patient to take control of a topic for discussion. It is a vehicle for genuine negotiation, for having a sensitive and purposeful conversation about change.

The worst way to use the agenda-setting chart is as if it is a checklist, controlled by the practitioner, in which the patient is asked to go through each behavior in turn. This loses the spirit of the task. We have found that the agenda-setting process is sometimes clouded by an issue which prevents it from being used constructively; the focus on changing lifestyle and encouraging the patient to take responsibility leads the patient to feel blamed for having the problem in the first place or at least blamed for not ensuring that progress is made. Observation that the patient is not engaged in agenda setting can be a clue that this problem is emerging. It is wise to understand the patient's feelings before continuing with the agenda-setting process.

Remember that visual aids like the agenda-setting chart are just that, and no more. If it does not feel comfortable to use it, don't! It is the general spirit of the encounter that is important.

Gobat et al. (2015) have explored what consensus there is about agenda setting in a clinical encounter, and consensus was obtained on six core domains: identifying patient talk topics, identifying clinician talk topics, agreement of shared priorities, establishing conversational focus, collaboration, and engagement. They propose using the terms "agenda mapping and agenda navigation." Research is ongoing into ways of specifying and observing best practice in these domains.

In the United Kingdom, there is a widespread use of "outcome stars" assessment tools, especially in community mental health settings and public health projects where many clients have complex needs socially and clinically. These tools (MacKeith, 2011) are designed to support and measure change and seem particularly useful when there are a host of issues to address and agencies to whom to signpost patients. With training and practice, practitioners can integrate their use of these with the consultation style discussed here to set relevant agendas while maintaining rapport.

STRATEGY 2. SINGLE BEHAVIOR — RAISE SUBJECT

In some circumstances, the practitioner has clearly identified one particular behavior that he or she wants to discuss. Where the setting is a particular clinic, for example, a smoking cessation clinic, the agenda is clear and explicit to both the patient and the practitioner; there is no need to worry about how best to raise the issue. Other situations are less straightforward and are most often in the context of a patient presenting with a particular symptom or disorder and the practitioner identifying a probable or certain link with a particular behavior. Alternatively, as a result of a health check, it may be that there is a single behavior that is clearly compromising the patient's optimum health.

Some practitioners do not believe that this is a particularly sensitive matter. They believe that it is their professional duty to raise a concern about risky health behavior and that not raising the issue would be to shirk this responsibility. Need this be an overriding assumption? Too many patients shift uncomfortably in their seats when a problem that has been raised by the practitioner "hits them in the face." Also, there are some research findings where interviews with patients suggest that they have strong views about this (see Stott and Pill, 1990). Of critical importance is the quality of the rapport between the parties. The professional responsibility is better seen as to raise an important health behavior issue in a manner and at a time such that the patient is likely to respond well.

WHAT TO AVOID

It is important to avoid raising the subject in a way that is perceived by the patient as patronizing and judgmental. Establishing a good rapport with the patient before raising the issue is important. Hopefully the days are gone when patients are met with comments like *I think we both know you've been a bit naughty about your…* [drinking, diet, etc.], *don't we?* or *You've brought this on yourself by smoking, haven't you?* Direct confrontation will in most cases elicit defensiveness.

If you have good rapport with someone, you can talk about any subject. Therefore, consider this as your first priority. Remember that you and the patient are both on the same side; you both have an interest in improving or maintaining his or her health. Be honest about your own agenda and invite the patient to express his or her own views on the subject. Here are several examples:

I've been wondering what is the most important thing we should concentrate on to improve your health at the moment. I think it would help you a lot if you could lose some of that excess weight. How does it seem to you? What do you think the priority should be?

Poor circulation is sometimes linked with or caused by smoking. I wonder if we could talk briefly about whether that might apply to you?

Have you ever considered whether getting more exercise might improve control of your diabetes?

How do you feel about the amount you drink?

Did you know that some people find that changing their diet can help improve heartburn? We could talk about that a bit if you're interested.

I'm concerned about your chest. I wonder how you feel about your smoking.

People who do little exercise are at greater risk of developing high blood pressure and heart problems. I wonder if you would be interested in talking through whether it might be worth your while to build some more physical activity into your life.

Be clear that your interest in the behavior is not because you disapprove of the patient doing it but because you think there may be some health benefits for them in changing. As a result, your inquiry and concern are legitimate and non-judgmental. At this stage, the subject is raised for discussion only, with the question of change still open.

THE DELICATE SUBJECT

There are some occasions when raising the subject can be undoubtedly difficult. There is no easy formula here, other than by taking time to establish a good rapport. Raising the subject of heavy drinking is a good example. A proud person who feels concerned about being stigmatized as an alcoholic can make things difficult for the practitioner concerned about his or her health. The mere mention of the word "alcohol" can produce immediate resistance. Put bluntly, as a Norwegian colleague has observed, undermine someone's self-esteem and he or she will resist your efforts (Tom Barth, personal communication). Under these circumstances, it seems easier to say what one should not do. Obviously, no reference should be made to words like "alcoholic," "drinking problem," or even "concern." Leave it up to the patient to reach this kind of conclusion. *Use of alcohol* is the safest phrase to use. If one encounters immediate resistance, this is a signal to change strategy.

In truth, an easy route through this problem has not yet been found; no simple strategy that will unlock a patient's willingness to talk, apart from conveying a genuine concern for the person and taking a matter-of-fact approach to the behavior. An example is a 45-year-old male patient who simply stopped eating in the face of enormous pressure at home. He had three children under the age of 5 years, one of whom had a serious respiratory problem. His partner was suffering from postnatal depression and dependence on alcohol. He was seriously sleep deprived and under stress at work. Eventually he was admitted to the hospital, passing blood in his urine. Through a series of complicated investigations, which included exploratory surgery, he remained passive and silent. One day, out of the blue, his anesthetist came to his bedside, closed the door, sat beside him, and asked what he thought might have caused his symptoms. The floodgates opened and the patient acknowledged his problems at home. He was discharged from the hospital soon afterward into the care of a psychologist. He said that this anesthetist was the only person who had seemed genuinely concerned about him as a person.

A productive way of building this kind of rapport is to ask about a typical day (see Chapter 6 for more detail on the Typical Day strategy). This immediately places a subject like alcohol use or unhealthy eating behavior in a normal context and protects you from becoming too investigative or confrontational (e.g., *How much do you really drink? Why do you drink?*). You might instead begin like this:

I really do not know a lot about you and the kind of life you lead. Perhaps we can spend a few minutes with you telling me about a typical day in your life, from beginning to end. If you like, as you go along, you can tell me where your diet, use of alcohol, and exercise fit in.

If you raise the subject and get the impression that the person is feeling threatened, it can be useful to give him or her time to think. This is fairly easy in a primary health-care setting, where continuity of care is a possibility. The person can come back and see you again. Back off in a nonthreatening way and come back to it later. Even in a hospital setting, we have found it useful to leave the person's bedside for a while and come back to the discussion at a later point in time. If a patient knows that your concern is genuine, and if you have a reasonable rapport between the two of you, the boredom of the hospital routine can make your return visit more interesting to the patient than you might expect.

Raby (1999) has summed up the challenges here, describing the "three Js" of raising the issue of drinking with elderly people:

- Make it clear it is your JOB. Make a link between the problems that are presenting and the possibility that alcohol may cause or exacerbate them.
- Show that you would not JUDGE them. Demonstrate that you understand the difficulties they experience and know that they are doing their best to get by.

- Remember not to JUMP ahead. Do not assume that because someone recognizes they have a problem, they are ready to change it.

KEY POINTS

- Taking time to establish rapport and show respect for the patient's right to choose is crucial.
- When there are several behaviors to discuss, the patient will be the one who knows the best place to start.
- Beware of focusing prematurely on one topic and on change.

REFERENCES

Gobat, N., Kinnersley, P., Gregory, J.W., Robling, M., 2015. What is agenda setting in the clinical encounter? Consensus from literature review and expert consultation. Patient Education and Counseling 98.7, 822–827.

MacKeith, J., 2011. The development of the Outcomes Star: a participatory approach to assessment and outcome measurement. Housing, Care and Support 14 (3), 98–106.

Raby, S., 1999. Not Born Yesterday: A Training Manual about Alcohol and Older People. Aquarius Action Projects, Birmingham.

Rollnick, S., Mason, P., 1992. Negotiating Behavior Change: A Selection of Strategies (Unpublished manual).

Stott, N.C.H., Pill, R.M., 1990. Advise yes, dictate no. Patients' views on health promotion in the consultation. Family Practice 7, 125–131.

Stott, N.C.H., Rollnick, S., Rees, M., Pill, R., 1995. Innovation in clinical method: diabetes care and negotiating skills. Family Practice 12, 413–418.

Assessing importance, confidence, and readiness

4

CHAPTER OUTLINE

INTRODUCTION

I'd love to give up smoking. I know it's bad for my health, the kids hate me smoking and it is becoming even more of a problem now that everywhere has become non-smoking. I just don't seem to be able to though. I've tried several times and the longest I last is about 3 weeks, so I've just about given up trying.

I could cut down my drinking any time if I really wanted to. When I went on that diet 2 years ago, I didn't drink at all for 6 weeks. But I don't see any need to cut down at the moment. I'm fit, I never get bad hangovers, and it doesn't interfere with my work or my family. If I saw the need, I would just do it.

59

It seems that some people cannot change and others do not want to. This chapter explores how to assess someone's readiness to change using these two dimensions and then how to respond, focusing on the element that is holding the patient back from change (Fig. 4.1 and Box 4.1).

It has been suggested above that a person's readiness to change (a more global concept) is influenced by his or her perceptions of importance and confidence, i.e., he or she can explain his or her stated position on a readiness to change continuum (see Chapter 2, Fig. 2.3, p. 30). Someone might be convinced of the personal value of change (importance) but not feel confident about mastering the skills necessary to achieve it (confidence). This applies to many smokers, especially now when so many people who used to smoke have given up, those still smoking tend to include a lot of people who feel themselves to be seriously addicted and locked into a smoking lifestyle. If they thought they could change they would have done

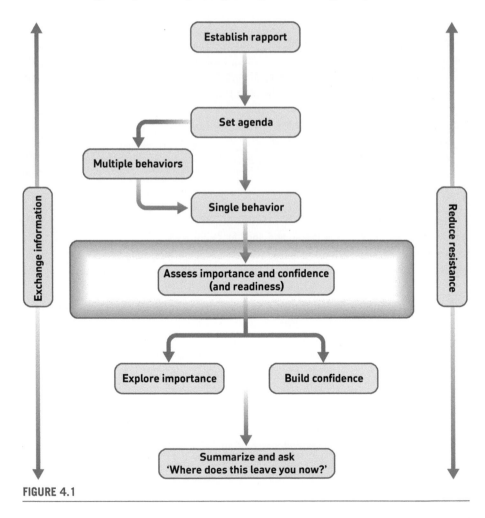

FIGURE 4.1

so already. Heavy drinkers, on the other hand, like the second patient above, can be quite different. They often have mixed feelings about the value of change (importance) but say that they could achieve this fairly easily (confidence) if they really wanted to. When it comes to changes in eating patterns, people often have relatively low levels on both dimensions.

Having agreed to talk about a particular behavior, there are a number of directions one could take. We have found that the assessment of importance and confidence is a useful first step, hence our decision to use this as the fulcrum for decision-making in this approach. Put simply, it helps you understand exactly how someone feels about change. It also helps you focus your limited time and resources on the most salient issue for each patient. We are not suggesting that this task needs to be carried out in every consultation. One might, for example, already know how a patient feels about change or at least have a strong intuition about this. You might decide to carry out another task, for example, exchanging information (Chapter 6), or use a strategy for exploring importance (Chapter 5). If the consultation is like a journey, assessing importance and confidence is one route that can profitably be taken.

Practitioners have different styles. Some people work in a less structured, more organic way, and their style is more conversational. Others prefer to have structured questions to ask and something of a format to follow. Below, you can see how to conduct this assessment in each style. In both cases, the assessment can take as little as 2—3 min.

WHAT TO AVOID

As our patients' health is our priority, it is easy to assume that it is theirs too. This can lead us to imagine that they share their health practitioners' conviction that it is important to change and that what is holding them back is that they do not know how best to do so. In turn, this can lead to an intervention based on practical advice with a touch of cheerleading thrown into boost motivation. Not all patients will be helped by such an approach.

So, we both know how important it is for you to lose weight. Let us find a diet that you think would work for you and book you into our slimming club to give you some moral support. I can see you do not look very enthusiastic, but we have had lots of success in helping people lose weight and you are really going to notice the difference in your health.

SCALING QUESTIONS: A STRATEGY FOR A MORE STRUCTURED APPROACH

> How do you feel at the moment about [change]? How important is it to you personally to [change]? If 1 was "not important" and 10 was "very important," what number would you give yourself?
>
> If you decided right now to [change], how confident do you feel about succeeding with this? If 1 was "not confident" and 10 was "very confident," what number would you give yourself?

Many health practitioners have experience of scaling questions like these, and patients may have experience in answering them in other contexts. They are frequently used in pain management and mood management and were first used in consultations about behavior change by De Schazer et al. (1986). They are adapted for our purpose here.

There are different ways of phrasing them, of course. It is helpful to clarify which end of the scale is which. The words *importance* and *confidence* seem to be the least ambiguous to express the ideas we are after. If, instead of asking how *important* something is, you ask *How motivated are you?*, the answer will sometimes be an amalgam of importance and confidence and be less useful in understanding the patient's position. One patient, in response to being asked *How motivated are you?* said *About a 5… I really want to but I don't know how possible it is!* Asking the questions as described above might have produced an 8 for importance and a 3 for confidence, which would have been much more helpful in deciding where to go next than the 5 which seemed to be an average of the two.

Sometimes, a patient will simply respond to the importance question by saying, *Very important*. In this case, you can move directly into the process of exploring importance as described in Chapter 5. A useful and obvious response is simply to ask, *Why?* This will invite the patient to speak in a positive way about the value of change and strengthen their resolve. These and other ways of responding are described in detail below.

A concept linked to importance is that of *wanting* to change or even *keenness* to change. The assessment question could be framed thus:

> How do you feel at the moment about [change]? How much do you want to [change]? If 1 was "not at all" and 10 was "very much," what number would you give yourself?

Scrutiny of the latter two questions reveals that they approach the more general concept of readiness, or motivation, to change. We have not suggested using this latter term in the assessment because, as noted above, some of our earlier work (see Rollnick et al., 1997) led to theoretical confusion about the meaning of the term *motivation*. In this particular assessment, we are interested in penetrating the patients' feelings and views about the costs and benefits of change, how they personally value change and whether it will, on balance, lead to an improvement in their lives, as distinct from the issue of their confidence to master the demands of this change.

In keeping with the meaning of the term *self-efficacy*, the focus, when asking about confidence, is not in a general sense of self-belief or self-esteem but in confidence about mastering the various situations in which behavior change will be challenged.

INTRODUCING THE ASSESSMENT

The patient should fully understand why you would like to use this strategy, and rapport should be good. It can be introduced thus:

I am not really sure exactly how you feel about [behavior or change]. Can you help me by answering two simple questions, and then can see where to go from there?

At this point, pause and deal with whatever response the patient makes. Sometimes, they do not allow you to get going and proceed to tell you how they feel! This is exactly what you want. Leave the assessment aside, and return to it if you are still confused.

If the patient seems disengaged, do not do the assessment. Attempt to raise the level of engagement first. Express curiosity. If your rapport is good enough, you can challenge the patient in a friendly way; for example,

Have you ever sat down with someone and told them exactly how you feel about [behavior or change]? I'd be interested to hear how it sounds from your perspective.

Or check it out with them:

In a discussion like this, it can be a mistake to jump too quickly to talk about doing this or doing that. I certainly don't want you to feel pressurized in any way. We could talk about something else.

A VISUAL AID CAN HELP

Even when doing a more formal assessment, the patient must be actively involved. You provide the structure, and the patient does the rest. If it looks or feels like a question and answer assessment session, you are falling short of the ideal.

* The assessment can be done verbally, using the questions above; the readiness rule can be downloaded from the website (http://evolve.elsevier.com/Mason/healthbehavior/) or photocopied from Appendix 3, or you can just draw lines on a scrap of paper by way of a visual aid!
* The spirit of this exercise is most important. You need to feel genuinely *curious*. It is not an investigation but an inquiry.

- The goal of the assessment is to work out which of the two domains, importance or confidence, should be your focus.
- The words one uses can be critical; for example, a smoker talking about quitting might respond differently to questions about her confidence to "give it a try," "stop for a week," or "never touch a cigarette again."

HOW THIS STRATEGY WAS DEVELOPED

This more standardized assessment procedure emerged from experimentation with smokers (Rollnick et al., 1997; Butler et al., 1999). The starting point was a need to develop a method that we could teach to family practitioners for use in consultations lasting 7−10 min. The goal was to find a way of conducting a quick psychological assessment of smoking, i.e., 2−3 min, which could lay the foundation for a conversation about change. Pilot work with a group of volunteer smokers began with a readiness to change continuum, hoping to use this as a guide to the choice of strategy that the practitioner might use. Initially, the issue became confused by the fact that people placed themselves in similar positions on a readiness continuum while having very different needs. The choice of strategy was not immediately apparent from the person's stated readiness to change. When asked *why* they had put a mark on a given point on the continuum, it emerged that the conversations tended to embrace two topics, importance and confidence, as described in Chapter 2. It was then decided to assess these dimensions directly, and a single-page intervention method was developed, based on this assessment, which was used for training practitioners (Rollnick et al., 1997). It was later found that they subsequently used this assessment in everyday practice, and not just with smokers but in other behavior change discussions.

When used in consultations with other kinds of behavior change problems, very few patients have difficulty with the numerical scaling technique on which the assessment is based. Of course, this depends crucially on the specificity and relevance of the change under discussion. The more specific the change, the easier it is to understand the assessment. In essence, this assessment of importance and confidence is a structured and directive way of enabling patients to say how they feel about a particular change within a couple of minutes. Its orientation is patient-centered; it provides a platform for responding to the domain defined by the patient as being in greatest need of attention. The decision where to go next within each domain is dealt with in Chapter 5. The focus here is merely on assessment.

A MORE CONVERSATIONAL APPROACH

The assessment can also be done informally. The following example illustrates the conversational process of unraveling which dimension is of greatest concern to the patient; in this case, in a conversation about exercise. An informal assessment of importance and confidence is shown below:

Practitioner: So, we have identified that you get very little exercise since your promotion to an office-based job, and consequently you have put on some weight. You also find the new job stressful and could do with a way of letting off steam. How do you feel about organizing some sort of physical activity for yourself now that you are not in a physically demanding job?

Patient: Well, I can see the need. I don't like feeling so unfit and I've never had such a belly on me in my life! I can't see myself paying out good money to go to a gym just to pump iron for the sake of it though. When I was loading trucks and so on, there was a purpose to it. I never stick with things I don't think are useful.

Practitioner: So you like being active if you're achieving something that's important to you. Have you ever been into sports? Ball games?

Patient: Not really. Although I used to be strong, I was never much good at the skill side, and games are not much fun if you're no good at them. It's hard to think what I could do that would, like you say, help me to let off steam and keep me in shape. I'd like to find something though.

It quickly becomes clear through a short conversational exchange that the patient understands and believes in the importance of change but will need some help to think creatively about how to go about it. He has no confidence that he would be able to pursue the solutions he can see at present.

It is useful to adopt a curious manner during this process, as this reflects your genuine interest in how the patient really feels. It is not a question and answer session over which the practitioner has complete control, but rather a matter of asking the patient to paint a picture. The practitioner is sitting back and allowing the patient to do most of the talking, leaving silences if necessary.

WHAT TO TALK ABOUT NEXT: IMPORTANCE OR CONFIDENCE?

The outcome of this assessment is sometimes clear. The patient has little concern about one dimension and the obvious difficulty lies with the other one. It is then a matter of deciding what strategy will help this person to either explore importance or build confidence. A menu of options within each dimension is provided in Chapter 5.

Sometimes it is not clear, or both dimensions appear salient. Here, one enters a labyrinth comprising the world of *can I, should I, will I, won't I?*, often not merely connected to behavior change but tied up with other personal matters:

I'd like to lose weight, but eating gives me such comfort. There's sometimes a hollow feeling in my stomach, when I get anxious or cross, the stress just gets too much. Then after eating so much, I feel disgusted with myself. It will be really difficult to stop this.

Habits can be complex, and difficult to change. Under circumstances like the above, practitioners clearly need to lower their sights if the contact time is brief. Being too ambitious is probably the biggest mistake to make, often taking the form of premature action talk: *Why don't we try to take things one step at a time, and start with…?* Resistance is a likely outcome. One possibility is that the discussion returns to agenda setting and moves on to another issue. The practitioner should ultimately use the patient as the guide for deciding whether to focus on importance or confidence.

The following guidelines are suggested for deciding whether to focus on importance or confidence. Practitioners should bear in mind, however, that there is no blueprint for decision-making, only aids for what is often an intuitive judgment.

- If the importance level is depressed, focus on this if at all possible.
- Focus on the lower number, importance or confidence, particularly if there is a large discrepancy between them.
- If they are approximately equal, start with importance.
- If they are both very low, lower your sights. Were you wise to focus on this behavior change in the first place? Consider the possibility that some other issue might be more relevant. Share this observation with the patient. Try to reach some agreement about exactly how the patient is feeling. Within each of the sections on importance and confidence below, it is always worth remembering that one option is to do little more beyond this assessment.

IS IT EASIER TO BUILD SOMEONE'S CONFIDENCE THAN TO CONVINCE THEM OF THE IMPORTANCE?

Many practitioners assume that confidence-building is easier to talk about, perhaps because this is congruent with a culture of action-oriented professional practice in health-care settings. This can even take the form of viewing motivational problems as confined to the issue of importance, as if confidence-building is somehow free of these difficulties. This can lead one into a trap; importance is viewed as complex, whereas confidence is viewed as a simpler practical matter of encouraging and helping with strategies for making the change. When talking about confidence-building, you feel you can get down to the real business of behavior change, apparently free of the delicate dance around the forces of resistance and motivation. Armed with this kind of understanding, a dash into advice-giving is usually just around the corner, and the response of the patient to suggestions about trying this or that action plan is predictable: *Yes, but I've tried that, and it doesn't work because…* Motivational problems can arise when talking about either dimension; for example, *I could if I wanted to, but…* (importance), or *I want to, but…* (confidence). There is no reason to believe that one dimension is essentially simpler to talk about or to "fix" than the other. Ambivalence about change can surely arise because of concerns about either or both.

FOUR STRATEGIES FOR ASSESSING READINESS TO CHANGE

There can be situations where it is useful to assess readiness, either instead of or in addition to importance and confidence. It can be a useful platform for taking the discussion a step further. This more global dimension is viewed more as something to be aware of on an ongoing basis throughout the consultation, not necessarily something to be assessed. It often provides an explanation for resistance if you overestimate the patient's general readiness to change (see Chapter 7).

Four assessment strategies are noted below:

- Open questions
- Scaling questions
- Readiness rule
- Little faces chart

The readiness rule is described in some detail, although it is important to note that the guidelines for it apply equally well to the other methods of assessment. The assessment of readiness is an ongoing process, not a one-off task, and it involves conversation and reflection.

Be specific. Readiness to do what? Usually, but not always, one is talking about a specific behavior. It is useful to be clear about this, and if you are not sure, check this with the patient. For example, taking the case of smoking, there is a difference between each of the following: readiness to talk about it, starting to cut down, experimenting with nicotine replacement therapy, setting a quit date. Each of these could be a useful topic for discussion.

WHAT TO AVOID

There are at least three ways in which our own attitudes can get in the way of this process. First, we can be so keen to improve people's lives that we forget they may be pretty content overall (even if we would not be, if we were them!). We want them to be ready to change, so we continue as if this is the case.

Second, we can take an "all-or-nothing" view of readiness: *Do you want to do this or not?* We forget how ambivalent people or "contemplators" are, swinging between wanting to change and not wanting to do so.

Third, we can become cynical, especially when under pressure, and write off those who seem unmotivated on the surface, without taking time to explore further.

FORMAL VERSUS INFORMAL ASSESSMENT

This assessment, like that of importance and confidence, can be done informally or explicitly. Below, we introduce a readiness rule and a little faces chart, both of which we have found useful in clinical practice. Of course, there is nothing to stop a practitioner from developing a similar practical tool divided into different stages or, indeed, built around the concepts of importance and confidence. Practitioners, like patients, have their preferences, and care should be taken not to view any piece of technology as comprising standard practice for all encounters.

In summary, people vary in their readiness to change their behavior; if you jump ahead of a patient, for example, by giving advice when he or she is not ready to change, resistance will be the outcome and your time will have been wasted. Your goal is to understand patients' degrees of readiness to change and to help them to move forward toward decision-making if they see this as worthwhile. Remember, readiness to change fluctuates between and within consultations.

STAGE BASED OR CONTINUUM?

If you do want to assess readiness, should you do this using the notion of stages or that of a continuum? Do people move between discrete stages or is it a seamless continuum of readiness for change? It is not clear which approach is more useful to practitioners. We have heard good arguments for each. A stage-based assessment appears to be clear and simple for both practitioner and patient, although questions have been raised about its scientific validity for matching interventions to patients (West, 2006). For practitioners new to this construct, the notion of stages can be very useful. As DiClemente and Prochaska (1998) have repeatedly reported, many behavior change efforts have been restricted to an action-oriented approach when most patients are not at this stage in the first place. Use of stage designations can be good for highlighting this kind of problem. We have discussed this in more detail in Chapter 2.

On the other hand, we all know that people jump in and out of stages. In fact, it is as if patients have different "voices" in their minds at any one time, representing different stages. This is particularly true for people designated as "contemplators." A mood of concern and optimism about change can swing to one of defensiveness and defiance in a matter of seconds. Practitioners, for their part, can become part of this conflict. Speak to them in one way, such as in a slightly coercive manner, and a resisting precontemplator's voice will emerge. Speak to them in another way, and a more optimistic voice can emerge. Thus, the apparent stage of change "in" the patient is the product of the interaction with the practitioner. This added complexity can render a stage-based assessment, particularly if viewed as a fixed, almost trait-like quality, oversimplified. It is for this reason that we generally find a continuum-based approach to assessment and strategy selection to be more fluid and easier to fit into a conversation.

For these purposes here, a "rough and ready" guide to how the patient is feeling about change is needed so that the intervention gets going in a way that is likely to be received with interest rather than resistance. As we go along, the practitioner can adjust the intervention as the patient's engagement and readiness for change shifts, so below is a look at strategies and visual aids to support this process. One visual aid uses stages and the other a continuum; both can be downloaded from the website (http://evolve.elsevier.com/Mason/healthbehavior/) or photocopied from Appendices 3 and 5.

STRATEGY 1. OPEN QUESTIONS

The easiest method to use is to ask simple *open questions* and then follow the patient's response carefully. For example,

How do you really feel about...? How ready are you to change?
People differ quite a lot in how ready they are to change their... What about you?
Some people don't want to talk about drinking at all, others are unsure, and some don't mind at all. How do you feel about this?

STRATEGY 2. SCALING QUESTIONS

One can also use a numerical scaling method; for example,

If 1 is "not ready" and 10 is "ready," what score would you give yourself?

Here, one can follow the response with similar questions to those outlined in detail in Chapter 5, where we look at how to respond to the assessment of importance and confidence. For example,

You gave yourself a score of X. Why are you at X and not [a lower number]?
You gave yourself a score of X. What would have to happen for you to move up to [a higher number]?

STRATEGY 3. READINESS RULE

A third method is to use something like the readiness rule (Fig. 4.2).
Introduce the assessment (the rule or a line on a piece of paper). For example,

How ready to change [behavior] are you? Where are you on this rule? Are you here [pointing to right-hand end], ready to change, or are you more toward the middle or the left-hand end?

Elicit the patient's judgment. If this is hampered by lack of information, ask the patient if he or she would like more information. Remember that this task might

Not ready		Unsure		Ready

FIGURE 4.2

A readiness rule.

Adapted from Stott et al. (1995), Family Practice 12, 413–416, Fig. 2, Oxford University Press, with permission of the publisher.

generate quite a lot of discussion. Do not rush this process, as it is crucial to decision-making.

Consider the next step. In general, if the patient appears unready, your only viable strategy might be to turn to information exchange to ensure that they have access to all the facts they need to continue to think about the issue (Chapter 6). If there is some readiness to at least consider change, try to work out whether you need to assess importance or motivation. If this is obvious, an appropriate strategy within either of these domains should be useful.

Watch the patient. Readiness to change fluctuates, particularly in the right-hand half of the continuum. Monitor this throughout the consultation. When people describe themselves as being on the right-hand end of the continuum, do not push them into decision-making. Remember that the consultation does not have to end with their having gone through the door saying something like *Yes, I'll definitely do something about it*. Even a decision to think about it can be a useful conclusion.

STRATEGY 4. LITTLE FACES CHART

Fig. 4.3 shows four little faces, each with a speech bubble containing a stage of change. This can be downloaded from the website (http://evolve.elsevier.com/Mason/healthbehavior/) or photocopied from Appendix 5. Show it to the patient and ask them which face they identify with most strongly. If they cannot choose because they identify in some ways with two or three faces, ask an open-ended question to get them to elaborate (*Tell me more about how you fit in somewhere between those two*) so that you can better understand their position. This pictorial version has been found to give a helpful and quick estimate of readiness to change (Rollnick et al., 1992; Mason, 1997). It has been designed to be, as far as possible neutral as to ethnicity or gender but you could draw your own to suit your patient group!

How one responds to a stage-based assessment is crucial. We do not suggest that practitioners think of a patient's identified stage of change as being linked with a specific intervention, for the reasons described in Chapter 2. Our starting point with a stage-based assessment would be to ask a patient why he or she is in one stage and not the previous one. This would open up the conversation for the patient to describe whatever basis there is for his or her interest in changing. We suspect that the conversation will inevitably turn to importance or confidence.

One can also use a stage-based assessment as a starting point for feeding back to the patient your understanding of how other people feel about change, using the principles for information exchange described in Chapter 6 and derived originally from the work of Miller and colleagues on the drinker's check-up (Miller et al., 1988; Miller and Sovereign, 1989). Thus, the expressed stage is used as the platform for letting patients interpret the personal meaning of their views in relation to others.

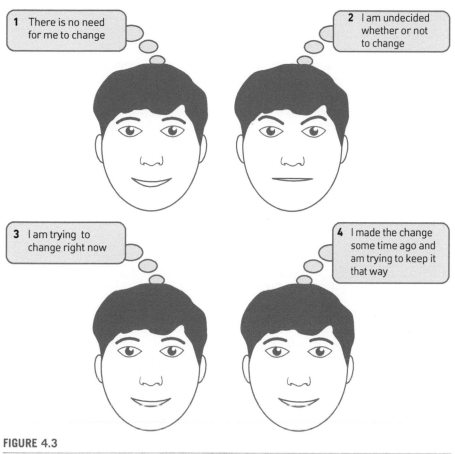

FIGURE 4.3

Little faces chart.

CONCLUSIONS: READINESS, IMPORTANCE, AND CONFIDENCE

If you were to assess all three dimensions, which kinds of patterns are likely to emerge? Another related question, and perhaps a more useful one, is to ask, at different degrees of readiness, what are the patterns that emerge on the other two dimensions? Researchers have looked at this second question, although this has taken the form of cross-sectional "snapshots" of people's expectations at different stages, rather than prospective studies of how they change as they shift forward through the stages. It does appear that the shift from the early stages of readiness to the later stages is associated with clear shifts in the perceived importance of change, i.e., as one might expect, change is perceived as more important as one becomes increasingly ready (Rollnick et al., 1996). There is apparently also a crossover effect in which the pros of change eventually outweigh the cons as people move through the stages (Prochaska, 1994). From the limited evidence, we have confidence issues that appear to become more salient in the later stages of readiness (Davidson, 1998; Rollnick, 1998).

From a clinical vantage point, these observations are important. If someone's readiness is low, the chances are that importance is the key issue. In the later stages of readiness, the person might be concerned about either importance or confidence. Indeed, one might even encounter a potentially bewildering overlap between importance and confidence in these later stages. It is in the melting pot of the contemplation stage, or to the right of the midway point on a readiness to change continuum, that the questions *Why should I?* and *How should I do it?* often collide. People often comment that being on the receiving end of such an exploration is really helpful in clarifying their own priorities and reluctances. The very process of a "no pressure" exploration seems to move them out of an impasse.

A CASE EXAMPLE OF AGENDA SETTING AND ASSESSMENT OF IMPORTANCE AND CONFIDENCE

Nurse: *Hello Mrs. Brown. How are you?* [Checks immediate problems and concerns]

Mrs. Brown: *I'm fine apart from being tired. The youngest boy has got a bit of a cough and I'm having to get up a couple of times a night so I'm not getting enough sleep just now.*

Nurse: *Do you want the doctor to see him?*

Mrs. Brown: *No. Thanks, he's got cough medicine and I think he'll be OK in a day or two, but I'll bring him in at the end of the week if he doesn't improve.*

Nurse: *Yes, do, if you're at all concerned. So, this appointment was to talk about your weight, wasn't it?* [Raises the issue]

Mrs. Brown: *Yes. You wanted me to lose some weight and I've been trying to slim on and off for years.*

Nurse: *So you've tried dieting.*

Mrs. Brown: *Yes, every diet you can name!*

Nurse: *We could either look again at diets, or look at how you could burn up more of the food you eat by being more active, or we could look at both.* [Invites patient to set agenda]

Mrs. Brown: *I think I probably know more about calories and diets than the doctor does! But I've never really made any effort to do any exercise when I'm dieting. I might think about that.* [Patient sets agenda]

Nurse: *How do you feel about becoming more active? Is it something you want to do? How important is it to you right now?* [Informal assessment of importance]

Mrs. Brown: *Well, when I was a girl I used to love sports — I was in the school hockey team and was never out of the swimming pool. Since the kids, I've let myself go a bit. I would like to feel fitter as well as losing some weight.*

I know I'd feel better about myself. I'd love to take the boys swimming now they're getting older too. [Patient gives information about her physical activity history and about how important it is to her to change]

Nurse: *So it's quite important to you.*

Mrs. Brown: *Very, now I come to think about it, but I've no idea whether it's realistic. Swimming would be the place to start but I don't know how I'd find the time, and I'm not sure I'd have the nerve to be seen in a swimsuit — the size I am now!*

Nurse: *So, you want to do it but you don't feel all that confident about it. If you decided right now to start swimming regularly, how confident do you feel about succeeding? If 1 was "not confident" and 10 was "very confident," what number would you give yourself?* [Formal assessment of confidence]

Mrs. Brown: *Less than 5 at the moment, partly because of the time and partly because I'd feel self-conscious. Perhaps if there was a time in the middle of the day when the kids are at school and nursery, and the pool is nice and quiet…? I don't know really.*

The nurse has structured the consultation clearly, but Mrs. Brown has had space to express her own interests and concerns. Having clarified that it is important to her to lose weight and to make physical activity a key behavior change toward this goal, it is obvious that confidence-building should be the focus. Note that if you count the words in this dialog, the nurse says less than Mrs. Brown. The nurse mainly asks questions and clarifies points. Mrs. Brown is talking herself toward an action plan, so far without needing any advice.

KEY POINTS

- It is helpful to consider motivation as a combination of placing a high value on doing something (importance) and believing in one's own ability to achieve it (confidence).
- We can understand a patient's attitude to behavior change best by inquiring about importance and confidence.
- Scaling questions are one helpful way of doing this.
- Inquiring about the more general readiness to change can help us know how best to move forward.
- Visual aids can help to facilitate assessment.
- This assessment is about the patient's attitudes and beliefs and is separate to assessment of the behavior itself (e.g., how much they drink, how much exercise they do).

REFERENCES

Butler, C.C., Rollnick, S., Cohen, D., Bachmann, M., Russell, I., Stott, N., 1999. Motivational consulting versus brief advice for smokers in general practice: a randomized trial. British Journal of General Practice 49, 611–616.

Davidson, R., 1998. The transtheoretical model: a critical overview. In: Miller, R.W., Heather, N. (Eds.), Treating addictive behaviors, 2nd edn. Plenum, New York.

De Schazer, S., Berg, I., Lipchick, E., et al., 1986. Brief therapy: a focused solution development. Family Process 25, 207–222.

DiClemente, C.C., Prochaska, J., 1998. Towards a comprehensive, transtheoretical model of change: stages of change and addictive behaviors. In: Miller, W.R., Heather, N. (Eds.), Treating Addictive Behaviors, second ed. Plenum, New York.

Mason, P., 1997. Alcohol counselling services in general practice (part II) who uses them and how? Journal of Substance Misuse 2, 210–216.

Miller, W.R., Sovereign, R.G., 1989. The check-up: a model for early intervention in addictive behaviors. In: Loberg, T., Miller, W.R., Nathan, P.E., Marlatt, G.A. (Eds.), Addictive Behaviors: Prevention and Early Intervention. Swets & Zeitlinger, Amsterdam.

Miller, W., Sovereign, R.G., Krege, B., 1988. Motivational interviewing with problem drinkers: II. The drinker's check-up as a preventative intervention. Behavioural Psychotherapy 16, 251–268.

Prochaska, J.O., 1994. Strong and weak principles for progressing from precontemplation to action on the basis of twelve problem behaviours. Health Psychology 13, 47–51.

Rollnick, S., 1998. Readiness, importance and confidence: critical conditions of change in treatment. In: Miller, W.R., Heather, N. (Eds.), Treating addictive behavior, 2nd edn. Plenum, New York.

Rollnick, S., Heather, N., Gold, R., Hall, W., 1992. Development of a short 'readiness to change' questionnaire for use among brief, opportunistic interventions among excessive drinkers. British Journal of Addiction 87, 743–754.

Rollnick, S., Morgan, M., Heather, N., 1996. The development of a scale to measure outcome expectations of reduced consumption among excessive drinkers. Addictive Behaviours 21, 377–387.

Rollnick, S., Butler, C.C., Stott, N., 1997. Helping smokers make decisions: the enhancement of brief intervention for general medical practice. Patient Education and Counseling 31, 191–203.

West, R., 2006. Theory of Addiction. Blackwell, Oxford.

Exploring importance and building confidence

5

CHAPTER OUTLINE

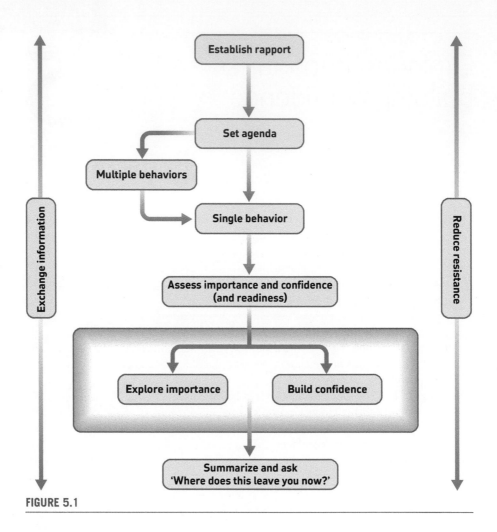

FIGURE 5.1

INTRODUCTION

Patient 1: Maybe I will quit one day, maybe I won't. Giving up is not really a problem. I've done it before without any problem whatsoever. I enjoy smoking and it doesn't seem to be doing me any harm. I know I shouldn't smoke in front of the children, especially little Maria with her bad chest. I don't suppose it sets a very good example. Still, my granny smoked 80 a day for 60 years and got run over by a bus while she was running across the road at the age of 85! I just enjoy smoking and it doesn't worry me.

Some patients attach a low importance to behavior change.

Patient 2: It's no good me trying to stop smoking. I know what you're saying is right. I ought to and I've tried lots of times but I've got no willpower. I last a couple of weeks and I'm back where I started.

Patient 3: I really can't see myself being able to remember to take this inhaler three times a day. It's easy to remember when my chest is bad. But when I feel better, I just forget completely although I know it's important to prevent my asthma attacks. I'm just not organized enough to do it.

Other people have so little confidence that it doesn't seem worth their even trying.

Having assessed the importance of change for patients and their confidence to put plans to change into action (see Chapter 4), you reach a critical junction. You need to decide where to go next and whether to focus on importance or confidence. This chapter explores a selection of strategies for working within either dimension. Usually, it is most productive to work on whichever seems to be lowest. For each of these topics, importance and confidence, a menu of strategies is given. Which one to use depends very much on the circumstances, your aspirations, and the needs of the patient.

THE DELICATE DANCE

In moving both within and between these dimensions, the practitioner will require all the skill and deftness of a dancer, leading a partner through a sequence of movements, simultaneously leading and being led, keenly alert to subtle threats to the synchrony of the partnership. Resistance from the partner is not met by force but by transforming the movement in a constructive direction, if at all possible. No amount of dedicated adherence to the strategies described below will be effective if this state of mind is absent. The strategies are merely aids to avoiding collision, like the steps one learns in a dancing class.

A certain degree of relaxation is required to maintain this spirit in the consultation. As noted earlier in this book, it is useful to develop a committed but curious state of mind when talking about behavior change. There is no sense in which the practitioner can be expected to have all the answers. Indeed, to work within the spirit of this approach, the practitioner must believe that these lie mostly within the patient.

FIVE STRATEGIES FOR EXPLORING IMPORTANCE

Five strategies are described in this section, all of which are options for exploring importance:

- Do little more
- Build on the scaling questions

- Examine the pros and cons
- Explore concerns about the behavior
- A hypothetical look over the fence

The range of strategies for exploring importance is best viewed as a menu from which one can be selected to suit your needs. Indeed, if you have time for development work, you might adapt these strategies and construct new ones more appropriate to your patient group.

Care should be taken not to view these strategies as techniques applied *to* or *on* patients. If this happens, it is an indication of detachment, which might damage rapport. The strategies are simply ideas for structuring a purposeful conversation. Their specificity should also not be misunderstood; this is intended as a guide, as a concrete reference point which is likely to minimize resistance. As noted from the outset, creative adaptation, not slavish adoption, should be the goal.

TAILORING THE STRATEGY TO THE PATIENT

Some of the strategies for working on importance are best used at fairly high levels of this dimension (i.e., with scores above 5/10 on the formal assessment). This applies particularly to exploring concerns; for example, if a patient does not see change as particularly important, and you use a strategy like exploring concerns, you could be in trouble! The patient will say, *What concerns?* The same logic applies to the hypothetical look over the fence. Others are safer or more widely applicable at all levels of importance: for example, scaling questions, and examining pros and cons. The strategies below are thus presented in ascending order of suitability to patients, from lower to higher levels of perceived importance.

Your use of words to describe different degrees of concern about a behavior can be critical. If a patient says, *My drinking is sometimes a problem*, and you respond reflectively with, *You think you might be becoming an alcoholic,* you could elicit resistance. If you give people a chance to talk, they will use a variety of words about change. You should watch out for these and match them as far as possible. Many of the strategies below start with a leading question that implies knowledge of how concerned the patient is about a behavior. Sometimes, however, one does not get a lead from the patient, and one has to take a deep breath and see what happens.

We have noticed that if one imagines a continuum of importance, from 0 to 10, different words are suitable at different points along this continuum. The wording *What is it you don't like so much about* [behavior]*?* is the safest bet, applicable for most people, provided that the level of reported importance is not 0. In ascending order, the following terms are appropriate, as the level of importance gets higher: *dislikes* or *less good things* (2–3/10 or above), *concerns* (6/10 or above) and *difficulty*, or *problem* (7–8/10 or above). When you are paying close attention to the way the patient is talking, their choice of words and body language, you will be able to choose intuitively the right way to phrase your inquiries.

STRATEGY 1. DO LITTLE MORE

If a patient's level of perceived importance is markedly low, particularly if accompanied by a low level of confidence, it might be advisable to close the discussion of behavior change and either turn to an issue they consider more important or end the consultation. How this is done is important. You could leave the patient feeling downhearted or even reluctant to come back and see you again. Consider saying something like:

Perhaps now is not the right time to talk about this? How do you feel?

You say you are unsure about what to do. I do not want to push you into a decision, it's really up to you. I suggest that you take your time to think about it.

I have met other people who have felt just like you do. Some, for good reasons of their own, decide not to do anything for the time being. Others do the opposite and make the change. You will be the best judge of when is the right time to consider change. Is there some other issue that feels more important to you?

Whatever you do, acknowledge the uncertainty, do not just leave the patient hanging in the air. If you are not sure what to do, ask the patient. For example, he or she might want to talk about it again on another occasion when other priorities have subsided: *I would like to talk about losing weight sometime but just now I'm so worried and stressed looking after my Mum while she's sick, I just can't think about it.*

Many practitioners faced with this situation are tempted to take a deep breath and simply provide information, seeing it as their professional responsibility to at least inform the patient of existing or potential risks. If this does not damage rapport, the approach seems understandable and justified. Chapter 6 discusses an approach to doing this.

STRATEGY 2. BUILDING ON THE SCALING QUESTIONS

This involves using a set of questions designed to understand and encourage the patient to explore the whole question of the personal value or importance of change in more detail. It builds on the numerical assessment described in Chapter 4 (adapted from work by de Shazer et al., 1986), although it can also be used in a nonnumerical form. Typically, having elicited a numerical judgment of importance, the set of simple questions noted below can open up a very productive discussion in which the patient is doing most of the talking and is thinking hard about change (see Rollnick et al., 1997).

You have already conducted an assessment of how important it is to the patient to change, and you have a given level, ideally a number, in mind although this is not essential. You can then ask open questions along the lines of: *Why so high? How can you go higher? What would it take to move you up a step? What number would you need to be on before you would give it a go?*

The aim of these questions is twofold: first, for patients to better understand their own points of view and to hear themselves speaking positively about change as something that might, at some point, be desirable or possible; second, for you, the practitioner, to better understand the key issues for patients and their current attitudes to change. To achieve this, ensure that the pace of the discussion is slowed down, and develop a genuine curiosity to know how this person really feels. You should listen to the answers to your questions, using techniques like reflection and other simple open questions to help patients express themselves as fully as possible. Your attention should not be on your own thought processes, *What should I say next?*, but as much as possible on the meaning of what the person is saying, *What exactly is it they are telling me?* Trust the process and the patient. Watch carefully for resistance because this is a signal that you are going too far or too fast.

Why so high?

Ask why he or she scored a given number and not a lower number. For example,

> *You said that it was fairly important to you personally to change [behavior]. Why have you scored 6 and not 1?*

The answers amount to positive reasons for change or in the jargon of motivational interviewing, *change talk* (Miller and Rollnick, 2012). For example,

> *I am at 6 and not 1 because I cannot go on like this forever.*

An obvious response is simply to ask *Why not?* or *What concerns you most about continuing as you are in the long term?*

Your task is now to elicit the range of reasons why the person wants to change. The pace should be slow, and simple open questions can be very useful. If the answers are obvious, elicit them and move on. If more complex, take your time trying to understand all the ramifications. If the patient gave the importance a level of 0 or 1, you would probably choose not to use this strategy! However, even with a 2 you might say:

> *So it's obviously not a high priority for you. However, you gave it a 2 and not a 1 or 0. I thought you might put it right down the bottom of the scale but you didn't. It sounds as if a little part of you attaches some importance to it? What's that about?*

Can you see how different it would be if you ask, *Why is it only as low as that?* This would invite negative statements about change and encourage patients to identify with the resistant side of the ambivalence.

Having elicited some change talk, explore it, reflect it, ask for more reasons why and ask for specific examples.

> *So you'd rate giving up smoking as a 5 on the importance scale because you'd like to save some money. [Reflection] Can I ask what you would like to spend the money on if you weren't spending it on cigarettes? [Asking for an example or elaboration]*

This is where the scaling questions become really powerful; not just as anssessment but as a way of focusing on the positive importance of change and, below, on the confidence that it could really be made to happen. Practitioners sometimes use the scaling questions enthusiastically as an assessment tool, forgetting that they are purely a subjective guide to how patients feel about something. They miss out on using them to actually help the patient discover and verbalize the various elements of their motivation and edge toward change.

How can you go higher?

A second kind of question moves in the opposite direction, up the scale from the number given by the person. For example,

You gave yourself a score of 6. So it's fairly important for you to change [behavior]. What would have to happen for your score to move up from 6 to 9? or How could you move up from 6 to 8 or even 9? or What stops you moving up from 6 or 7 at the moment?

Note that one can ask about either *your score* or just *you*. The second often feels better. In answering these questions, the patient opens up the possibility that change might be an option at some point, perhaps if things were a bit different. It also helps the practitioner to understand the obstacles or barriers to change.

Here is an example of dialog which illustrates that the key challenge for the practitioner is to carefully follow the patient's response, with further questions and reflective listening statements. In this example, the practitioner starts with the first kind of question described above: *Why so high?* and then simply follows the responses of the patient. It is not necessary in this example to move on to using the second kind of question: *How can you go higher?* The conversation flows quite naturally into that territory; what would make the person more motivated? Note how the use of a new strategy involves being quite directive to begin with; the practitioner offers a structure to the conversation.

Practitioner: [A few minutes into the consultation. Decides that the patient will respond to a quick assessment of importance and confidence.] *How do you really feel about taking more exercise? If 0 was "not important to you at the moment" and 10 was "very important," what number would you give yourself?*

Patient: [A short silence] *About 6.*

Practitioner: *And if you did decide now to take more exercise, how confident are you that you would succeed? If 0 was "not confident" and 10 was "very confident," what number would you give yourself?*

Patient: *About 8.*

Practitioner: *So if you decided to do it, you feel fairly confident, but you are not sure how important it is for you right now.*

Patient: *Well yes, that's about right.*

Practitioner: *You said it was fairly important for you, a score of about 6. Why did you give yourself 6 and not 1?*

Patient: [Initial silence] *I am at 6 and not 1 because I know I need to make my heart work harder in order to get it strong again. I understand the logic of that. If I had broken my leg, I'd do physio to get better again. Now that I have had a heart attack, I guess I should go back to my walking and swimming.*

Practitioner: *It will be good for you.* [Intonation as reflection rather than advice]

Patient: *Well that's what you people always say!*

Practitioner: *But you're not so sure.*

Patient: *No. Well, part of me wonders if I wouldn't be better resting up for a bit longer.*

Practitioner: [Decides to use information exchange. Becomes more directive.] *So getting well is your priority. Have you ever had a good talk about what happens in the heart after a heart attack?*

Patient: *Yes, sort of, but I don't understand…*

Note that the practitioner could have returned to the structure provided by the scaling question on a number of occasions: for example, *So your fear of damaging your heart is stopping you taking more exercise. Were it not for this, what score would you give yourself for wanting to get more exercise?* In this example, however, the scaling method was used as a springboard, not as a scaffold for the entire conversation. In other situations, it can be very useful to go back to the scale and the numbers.

You might wonder about the outcome of this kind of discussion. Where should it lead? It is unwise to generalize about this because it depends on the unique needs of the individual. The point is that simply talking about the importance dimension can help to clarify things. It might or it might not lead to firm talk about change. The question, *Why so high?*, invites the patient to spell out the reasons for change, which is more useful than their sitting listening to you doing that. It is best to follow the patient. If the discussion ends without action talk, simply summarize what has been said, offer whatever future support you can, and leave it at that. The aim of the consultation is not to get agreement or a decision to change but to support the patient on the journey toward deciding what to do. Exploring importance is just that — exploration.

STRATEGY 3. EXAMINE THE PROS AND CONS

Unlike Strategy 2, use of Strategy 3 does not have to be based on an explicit assessment of perceived importance. It is sometimes completely obvious that the importance of behavior change is an issue, and the only challenge is to decide what strategy to use to explore whether this importance can be increased at all. When it is preceded by a numerical assessment, this strategy is ideal when the score is around 5/10 on the scale. At 1/10, the patient might not perceive any costs associated with the behavior at all.

One aspect of the internal conflict (see Miller and Rollnick, 2012) focuses on the costs and benefits of both staying the same and change. A conflict like that described in Table 5.1 might arise. Whichever way the person turns, there are costs and benefits associated with each option, change or no change. This has been termed a *double approach—avoidance conflict*.

The different ways in which people experience this kind of conflict are not understood well enough. Certainly the experience embraces both psychological and social dimensions. In the addictions field, it has been well documented by Orford (2001). From excessive drinking, through gambling, to forms of sexual promiscuity, the intense battle between episodes of indulgence and restraint can render a person confused, elated, guilty, depressed, optimistic, and often enmeshed in conflict with others. It is therefore not surprising that alternatives to direct persuasion like motivational interviewing were first developed in the addictions field (see Miller, 1983). The potential for conflict with a counselor is great. Within a few minutes, a patient's mood can swing from defiance to remorse, from agreement about a problem to apparent denial of one.

In health care, we are not necessarily working with someone in the throes of a severe addictive problem or what Orford (2001) called an *excessive appetite*. It could be a much more common dilemma. Mood swings might not be so severe, and there is no reason to believe that overweight or even obese people walk around in a state of severe conflict. We simply do not know enough about how people facing behavior change feel. Clinical experience tells us that among the people seen in health-care settings where behavior change is discussed, the nature and extent of the conflict vary considerably. This variation occurs on a number of dimensions.

One of the most striking variations is in the breadth of the conflict. Some people are truly faced with the kind of multifaceted conflict described in Table 5.1. Others

Table 5.1 Ambivalence

Someone facing the apparent need to change their diet might feel thus:	
No change	Change
COSTS	**COSTS**
Feel ugly and unattractive	Will have to think about what to eat all the time
Difficult to buy nice clothes	Will have to give up my favorite junk foods
Greater risk of heart disease and diabetes	Healthy food is often expensive
Can not run around easily with the children	
BENEFITS	**BENEFITS**
Do not have to think about what to eat, can eat with the family	Feel good about achieving it
Can eat the food I really like	May feel fitter and be healthier
	If I lose weight, I will feel more attractive and confident, and be able to buy nice clothes
	Will be able to be more active

appear to be very uncertain about change, not because they are in conflict about the *status quo* but because one major issue or perceived cost of change predominates over all else. An example would be a back pain sufferer who would very much like to become more active but who feels reluctant to do some simple exercises because of a fear of causing further damage.

There is also variation in people's awareness of the conflict and whether they have spoken about it before. Smokers, it seems, are usually aware of the competing costs and benefits, excessive drinkers generally less so. Some patients have never spoken about their feelings and views before and leave one feeling privileged to be hearing an account for the first time. Yet we all know patients for whom this is all familiar territory, almost to the point where they are ready and waiting for the practitioner to open up this little black box. They know the contents, and they are ready with the answers that allow them to avoid consideration of change at this point in their lives.

An interesting dimension is the degree of emotional intensity involved. This varies across individuals and behaviors. Generalization would be unwise, as would a conclusion about whether it is better to encourage patients to explore these issues on an emotional or a cognitive level. Sometimes, the emotional expression of ambivalence can feel confusing for patients, and it is the articulation on a more cognitive level that seems clearer, more conscious, and more helpful. The opposite can also be true. It is probably best to let the patient be one's guide here, paying careful attention to resistance at all times. We have also found that as the patient makes a decision to change and ambivalence is resolved (at least temporarily), this is often accompanied by an emotional reaction. The person sighs deeply or even becomes upset. This can be most constructive, although the patient will obviously need commitment from the practitioner to look after him or her in an appropriate way.

Finally, there is often a distinction between short- and long-term consequences, with the former having a more powerful effect on decision-making than the latter.

A drink makes me feel better today although I will wake up tomorrow feeling rough.

Smoking feels good and seems to relax me now although I know it is dangerous to my health.

It feels better to be spontaneous and not to use condoms, although I know I am risking getting an infection at some point.

In summary, this aspect of ambivalence is not like an accountant's balance sheet: rigid and rational, consistent in structure. It is an individual conflict about the personal value of change, often riddled with unique perceptions and contradictions. As such, there are few grounds for dogmatism and generalization about its content.

WHAT TO AVOID

A patient may be experiencing this internal conflict as an argument he or she is having with him- or herself. We do not want to take sides in this argument. If the patient can give reasons for changing and reasons for not changing, we have to give due consideration to both. If we take the side of change, the patient is likely to respond with the other side of the argument to redress the balance. People can then easily end up talking themselves into not changing or digging their heels in against change.

Practitioner: If you continue being so inactive, your weight is going to keep going up and your risk of a heart attack is really quite high. I know you would feel much better in yourself if you did more and were fitter. [Takes the side of change]

Patient: But I'm far too busy to waste time going to gyms or running in circles round the park. One of my colleagues had a heart attack when he was out jogging last year and that put a lot of us off, I can tell you! I don't think exercise has anything to do with my weight anyway. We've always been big in my family. [Defends the *status quo*]

This strategy is best used in the consulting room. However, if time is short, you can ask the patient to do the work at home, using a blank copy of the balance sheet presented in Table 5.2; this can be downloaded from the website (http://evolve. elsevier.com/Mason/healthbehavior/) or photocopied from Appendix 6. It can take as little as 5–7 min to use or as long as an hour. If you have more time, use it and let the patient explain things as fully as possible. The most important first step is to ask the patient whether he or she would like to examine the pros and cons. For example,

Would you like to spend a few minutes talking about your…? Looking at what you like and don't like about it?

or

Sometimes it can be helpful to examine the pros and cons of…? Would you find it helpful to spend a few minutes doing this, or would you prefer not to?

Another approach is to present the balance sheet to the patient, for example,

Here is a drawing that might help us. You can see that, for all people who are unsure about change, there are pros *and* cons *of staying the same [present behavior], and then there's the other side, there are usually* pros *and* cons *of change as well. Have you ever thought about it like this? Would you like to spend a few minutes talking about it?*

Table 5.2 Balance sheet

No change	Change
Costs	**Costs**
Benefits	**Benefits**

Use of words is important here. The most common mistake is to use needlessly technical words like *costs* and *benefits*. Even the use of *advantages* and *disadvantages* can be difficult for some patients. *Pros* and *cons* are usually acceptable; we have used *good things* and *less good things* below. If possible, the use of *like* and *do not like* are ideal. Be careful not to use words like *problem* or *concern* unless the patient has used them. They often imply a greater degree of concern than felt by the patient and can generate needless resistance, particularly with those who are less motivated to change.

One key decision is whether to focus on the pros and cons of continuing with the current behavior pattern or pros and cons of changing or both. Note that the content of one side of the divide is often a mirror image of the other and that the distinction often breaks down in conversation with patients. However, asking questions from both perspectives can generate more information. Thus, talk about cons of smoking (e.g., feeling unhealthy) will quite naturally evolve into talk about pros of change (feeling fitter). However, we suggest that you take the following rough guidelines into account. Start with the current behavior if

- you don't know the patient very well
- the patient seems unclear about the issues or has not had the chance to talk about them in a nonthreatening environment
- the patient is some distance from the preparation stage, i.e., is not actively thinking about change
- the patient feels ashamed about the behavior

The pros and cons of the current behavior

Your role is to provide structure, listen carefully, and then summarize at the end. The patient's role is to explain to you how he or she really feels. Start with the positive, which will help with rapport building and place the behavior in a normal context. This can be a shock in some situations, particularly where the patient believes that the behavior is a problem or at least believes that you are convinced it is a problem. You can deal with this in a quite straightforward way by explaining that there must be benefits from the activity or behavior; otherwise he or she would not be doing it.

- Ask a question like: *What are the good things about* [behavior]? Elicit these and summarize if necessary. Your role here is simply to understand. Try not to ask questions that do not have a direct bearing on this picture and its meaning. Simple open questions can be very useful; for example, *Why is this? In what way? How exactly does this affect you? Tell me more about…*
- Then ask a question like: *What are the less good things about* [behavior]? Elicit these, one by one, taking as much time as possible; use simple open questions to understand exactly what the patient does not like about the behavior; for example: *What don't you like about…?* or *How does this affect you?*
- Summarize both sides of the no-change position, as succinctly as possible, with the same words as those used by the patient. This is a simple skill, but it does

require practice. One needs to do at least two things at the same time: listen very carefully and remember the exact key words used by the patient to describe the pros and cons.

THE PROS AND CONS OF CHANGE

This is useful if you think that the patient is ready to look over the "other side of the fence."

- Ask a question like: *What might be the good things about change?* Elicit these and summarize, if necessary.
- Then ask a question like: *What might be the less good things about change?* Elicit these, slowly and carefully.
- Summarize both sides of the change position, as succinctly as possible, using the patient's own terminology.

STRATEGY 4. EXPLORE CONCERNS ABOUT THE BEHAVIOR

This strategy focuses solely on the costs of the current behavior or situation. One can only use it, with its emphasis on the word *concern*, if the patient appears concerned. Misjudgment of this, i.e., overestimating the level of concern, will result in resistance. Otherwise, it is ideal for helping the patient to take time to express exactly what the issues are. Its use will automatically generate *change talk*. This strategy was developed in health promotion consultations with heavy drinkers (see Rollnick et al., 1992). It focuses on one side of the ambivalence chart in Table 5.2, i.e., on concerns about the *current behavior*. Of course, one could also use it to examine concerns about *change*.

Two principles guide the use of this strategy: First, the patient, not the practitioner, expresses the concerns and second, once the patient has reached the end, the practitioner asks some key questions about the possibility of change. Your role is to provide structure, listen carefully and then summarize at the end. The patient's role is to explain to you how he or she really feels. To start off, either of the following two questions would be useful: *What concerns you the most about your* [behavior]*?* or *What concerns do you have about* [behavior]*?*

Then simply follow the patient's description, attempting to understand exactly why he or she feels this way, under what circumstances, and so on. Take your time. Go through any other concerns he or she might have. Exchange information, if appropriate, but try not to wander off task. Your role is to help the patient paint a picture of exactly why he or she is concerned. Then, summarize these concerns for the patient and ask about the next step.

Do this in a gentle and nonconfrontational way: *Where does this leave you now?* This kind of question is deliberately phrased in neutral terms. The patient can either move toward or away from a decision to change. A question which explicitly asks about change, *Now you've told me about your concerns, how do you feel about change?*, can be useful but carries the risk of the patient feeling pushed too far.

Taking a realistic look at current behavior can increase motivation to change by clarifying or enhancing concerns. Keeping a diary for a day or a week can be a useful way of understanding behavior and planning change. A patient who sees him- or herself as a moderate drinker might be surprised by the number of glasses poured from the wine bottle or the number of beer cans taken from the refrigerator. Similarly, someone who believes he is a healthy eater might underestimate the number of bags of chips and other snacks eaten between meals. In summary, diary-keeping clarifies when, how much, and in what context the behavior occurs.

It is less helpful to impose diaries on patients; this should form part of a joint decision and interest into examining the behavior in question. Care should be taken to establish a realistic time frame for keeping the diary that seems manageable to the patient.

Keeping a diary can serve other purposes: for example, in monitoring progress once the patient has decided to change.

STRATEGY 5. A HYPOTHETICAL LOOK OVER THE FENCE

This is yet another way of examining the implications of behavior change. We have not developed it in any depth because its application seems mostly to be a simple repetition of one half of the pros and cons strategy described above: that which concerns change. It is highlighted here as a separate strategy mainly because of the way in which it is introduced to the patient and because of the hypothetical tone of the conversation as a whole. It seems best used at relatively high levels of perceived importance, i.e., at levels of the numerical equivalent of 7/10 or more, although this judgment is based on clinical speculation alone.

At the risk of stating the obvious, the higher the level of perceived importance, the more someone will be thinking about change, about what it might be like on the other side of the fence. However, even at these high levels, change can be difficult to talk about. We think this is because as the patient's overall readiness increases, so he or she quite naturally has an almost simultaneous urge to back off. You ask about change, even in the form of an open-ended question: *How do you feel about change?,* and he or she articulates the arguments against it. Sometimes this arises from a genuine desire to express concerns about change (described in motivational interviewing as "sustain talk") which must be listened to and certainly not argued against with a *Yes, but…* response from the practitioner. At other times, however, one gets the feeling that this is merely a "back-off" voice, repeating well-worn private arguments for staying the same. Gauging the difference between these two possible reasons for expressing concern about change can be very difficult.

It may be possible to lift both oneself and the patient out of this confusion by deliberately making the discussion hypothetical. This avoids the risk of a patient feeling threatened and using this "back-off" voice. Both parties are taking a detached and curious look at what would happen. The patient is free to roam and speculate, without any pressure to make a decision in the consultation.

The opening sequence in the example below is one way of introducing this strategy. The exchange which follows highlights the tone of the discussion; this is explicitly curious and hypothetical throughout and then ends with a reassurance that the conversation was not meant to push the patient toward change, only to encourage open discussion about what it might be like.

The overlap between importance and confidence issues (see below) is highlighted in the use of this strategy, particularly when it is used at fairly high levels of importance; what can tilt the balance in favor of change and make it feel more worthwhile is a clear vision of being able to achieve it. In this sense, this strategy is suited to dealing with both importance and confidence issues. It is placed here merely as a matter of convenience. Here is an example:

Practitioner: So you are not sure that it's a good idea to try to change your diet.

Patient: That's right.

Practitioner: Why don't we just imagine for a moment that you *did* make this change. How would you feel?

Patient: [Laughs] Not very excited.

Practitioner: You fear that you might get less enjoyment from food.

Patient: Exactly, yes, because I enjoy fried food.

Practitioner: You would have to deprive yourself.

Patient: Sometimes I would, yes, but would I have to stop fried foods altogether?

Practitioner: I'm not sure. I imagine that you might have quite a lot of freedom, to start slowly, to cut back a little, to find other foods that you like. You would have to decide what's best for you and what would get the results that you want.

ETHICAL REMINDER

It is when dealing with the importance dimension that you can often run into ethical difficulties. You might very much want the patient to change, and you unwittingly push him or her toward this. Perhaps even worse, you consciously use a subtle "technique" for motivating change. To do this would be to violate the spirit of this kind of negotiation. Here are suggestions for protecting yourself and the patient:

- Be honest with the patient about what you are planning.
- Watch for resistance. When you go further than patients want, they will resist.
- Understand the patient's point of view. Empathy is your protection. Let the patient be your guide.
- "If in doubt, leave it out." There might be very good reasons not to change.

If you are unsure whether the person has a grasp of the information needed to make an informed choice check it out; see Chapter 6 for guidance for doing this while maintaining the spirit of the consultation.

A CASE EXAMPLE OF EXPLORING IMPORTANCE

Practitioner: So, it's not very important to you, right now, to cut down your drinking. On a scale of 1−10, you said you would only give it a 4. You obviously enjoy a drink. Tell me some more about how it fits into a typical day for you.

Patient: Well, I only drink in the evenings. I've never been much of a lunchtime drinker. Most days, I have a few beers in the club after work and then get a take-away on the way home. Often I'll have a whiskey as a nightcap while I watch some late night television. [This is a much shortened version of the Typical Day strategy described in Chapter 4.]

Practitioner: So what is it you enjoy about a drink in the club after work? [Elicits the pros of the current behavior]

Patient: It helps me unwind and there's a regular crowd in there to have a laugh with. It passes the time too. Since I've been on my own, I'm not so keen to go back to an empty house.

Practitioner: I can see that. And the nightcap?

Patient: That's partly habit and partly to make sure I sleep well.

Practitioner: I can see that there are lots of good things for you about drinking. Are there any not so good things? [Elicits cons or change talk]

Patient: Well, it takes up all my spare cash, but as far as I'm concerned, that doesn't matter as long as I'm enjoying myself.

Practitioner: [Senses a little resistance so backs off instead of asking directly about any other cons] So, it helps you relax, pass the time and sleep well. You're not concerned that it takes up your spare cash because you enjoy it, so in that sense, it is worth it. [Summarizes] So why did you rate cutting down as high as 4? Perhaps it's not even a 4 just now? [Why so high?]

Patient: Maybe not. Although a couple of the lads in the club have cut down lately on their doctor's advice. I'm fit as a fiddle but it did make me wonder whether I might be doing myself some damage without knowing it. I wouldn't want to make myself ill and I'd think twice if I thought I was. [Unasked, gives a response to *What would have to happen for you to seriously consider changing?*] How would I know if I was doing myself any harm? There isn't any way of knowing I suppose?

Thus there is an opportunity to go on to exchange information, perhaps explore concerns about health related to drinking and consider the pros of change.

FIVE STRATEGIES FOR BUILDING CONFIDENCE

Five strategies are described in this section. All of them have been devised to help build confidence:

- Do little more
- Build on scaling questions
- Brainstorm solutions
- Past efforts: successes and failures
- Reassess confidence

A menu of strategies was suggested above for exploring importance. A similar approach has been used here for deciding what strategy to use when helping patients with confidence issues. Choose a strategy that fits with the way the patient describes his or her lack of confidence. These strategies are not completely separate from one another. They are overlapping, being different ways to approach the subject of confidence-building.

A patient was recently heard to say something that seemed like an echo of so many other consultations: *I need to lose weight. I understand why. I know what to do, and why I should do it. But tell me, why is it that I have so little motivation?* Some patients really want to change. It is important to them to do so. However, they feel pessimistic about the success of such a venture. The remainder of this chapter describes strategies for building confidence to succeed. These strategies provide a framework for something which is pervasive in medical consultations and counseling sessions: helping people with practical solutions to their difficulties, building their confidence so that they leave the discussion thinking, *Yes, I can do that.* The frequency with which this activity occurs lies in sharp contrast to the absence of teachable strategies for improving its effectiveness (a similar situation to that other common activity in consultations, information exchange; see Chapter 6). It could be argued that we do not need such strategies because we know how to do it; we give them good advice but one has only to observe oneself or other consultations to see how readily such talk can descend into an unconstructive dialog. It is a simple activity to conceptualize, apparently, but difficult to succeed with. All too often, the patient says, *Yes, but I've tried that and it doesn't work because…*

Self-efficacy refers to a person's confidence in his or her ability to make a specific change in behavior. This will vary across situations. For example, a smoker might feel very confident about resisting temptation to smoke at work but less so when socializing with friends, and so on. Someone struggling with assertiveness might feel able to stand up for him- or herself when taking a faulty article back to a store but less able to stand up to his or her aged mother.

It is in the world of doing, and watching others making changes, that people are successful: not just in the world of talking about doing, as occurs in the consulting room. This accords with clinical experience; we know we are talking about most important matters with patients, i.e., their confidence to make changes, yet we have to bear the frustration of being one step removed from the world in which the patient's ability is to be tested. We all know patients who say, *Yes, I know what I have to do, but I just can't succeed. I keep failing.* Bandura's work (1977) points to the importance not of some mysterious quality called willpower but of levels of skill and ability and actually working on changes in the real world.

> *People often have the knowledge and skills to make desired changes once they have decided to do so (Arkowitz et al., 2008).*

For practitioners, the following practical guidelines can be derived from the work of Bandura and others (see, e.g., Egan, 1994):

- Self-efficacy is not an all-or-none quality. As it varies across situations, one can provide encouragement and praise for those situations where it is high and help the person look at different approaches for improving self-efficacy in situations where he or she feels less confident.

- Doing is the best way to enhance self-efficacy. Build as many bridges as you can between the consulting room and the patient's everyday life (e.g., bringing a partner to the next consultation, returning for brief meetings, patient-held records).
- People need to have skills to succeed. Sometimes these lie dormant; sometimes they need to be built up. They are seldom either entirely present or totally absent.
- Feedback should be provided about deficiencies in performance, not deficiencies in the person (Egan, 1994).
- People learn by modeling themselves on others, hence the value of talking about friends and patients who have succeeded, attending self-help groups, and so on.

A more general feeling of low self-esteem and helplessness often underlies poor self-efficacy to make more specific changes. Furthermore, what manifests as a psychological "problem" of low self-esteem often has strong social origins: *There's no chance of finding a job. So I can't move out of the damp flat. I haven't got the money to enjoy myself, and every time I try to change I fail. Now you say I must get my weight down.*

The strategies described below are not meant to be counseling strategies for dealing directly with low self-esteem and helplessness. Rather, they deal with more specific changes in self-efficacy about behavior change. Sometimes, however, you will find that if you can encourage someone to look at small changes, and if that person succeeds, these changes often have a bearing on gradually improving self-esteem. If not, simply acknowledging the way a person feels can start off a process of reversal of low self-esteem, particularly if you can offer further support.

GOALS, STRATEGIES, AND TARGETS

We use different terms to describe people's efforts to change behavior. Goals, strategies, and targets are among the most widely used. Without wishing to become immersed in precise definitions, it can be useful to note the way in which the use of terms like these varies from the general to the specific. They can be likened to signposts on a journey. This might start with talk about a general *goal* or outcome being aimed at, which provides an answer to the question, *What change would you like to make?* Usually this refers to behavior change, although the goal of losing weight provides an interesting exception; losing weight is an outcome of behavior change rather than a behavior as such.

The journey often continues with talk about *strategies*, and when one becomes even more specific, about *targets*. Discussing strategies and targets thus provides answers to the question, *How are you going to achieve this goal?* Thus, numerous strategies might be considered in pursuit of a single goal, and in turn, numerous targets might be considered in pursuit of a single strategy. No wonder, then, that talk about behavior change can be complex!

Table 5.3 Goals, strategies and targets: from the general to the specific

Goal	→	Strategy	→	Target
Lose weight		**1.** Eat less fatty food		**1.** Cut out fried potatoes **2.** No red meat during the week **3.** No full-fat milk
		2. Start eating new food		**1.** Fruit once a day
		3. Replace certain foods		**1.** Baked potatoes or rice instead of fries **2.** Fish instead of meat at weekends **3.** Fruit instead of dessert 3/7 days **4.** Poached egg or beans on toast instead of bacon for breakfast
		4. Get more exercise		**1.** Walk to work whenever possible **2.** Arrange sport or dancing once a week **3.** Use the stairs instead of the elevator

Table 5.3 is not intended to show the ideal weight loss plan. Rather, it simply shows the range of potential topics for discussion in the consulting room, which move from the general to the specific. It is this movement that is important to note, not the precise definition of the terms *goals*, *strategy*, and *target*. *Get more exercise* might be a goal for one person but a strategy toward another goal for someone else. The number of options for change increases as one becomes more specific.

Table 5.3 gives rise to a number of implications for practice. First, there is no point in talking about a target if the goal being pursued is not clear. Ideally, the patient should choose this goal. Less obvious is how often practitioners make the mistake of talking about a target without first checking whether another strategy might be more attractive to the patient; one that would give rise to an altogether different choice of targets. Using weight loss as the example again, there are so many options, admittedly some healthier than others, that it is worth checking which the patient would feel most confident about to begin with. Among the guidelines to emerge from this simple framework are the following:

- It is a good idea to get as far through this sequence as possible. *The more specific the target, the better.* Having said this, a premature leap to specificity can be dangerous.
- The patient is the expert in what is likely to work for him or her.
- There are often more options for change than patients realize. Opening up the discussion to examine alternatives and encouraging patients to choose those which they feel most confident about are useful activities (see Strategy 3 below).
- There is a lot of scope for providing information to patients about the wide range of options available and about the experiences of other patients.
- Levels of confidence to succeed will vary across and within an array of strategies and targets. Reassessing confidence can thus be used as an important guideline in selecting options (see Strategies 2 and 5).

- A patient's level of self-efficacy to achieve a specific goal will be determined by his or her confidence to achieve a wide array of smaller targets, like those described in Table 5.3.

STRATEGY 1. DO LITTLE MORE

Most decisions to change do not take place in the consulting room. The patient does not necessarily need to set specific targets in conversation with you. It might be enough to simply raise the issue, mention the possibility of taking action, and leave it at that. If continuity of care is possible, this is often a very good starting point, much better, for example, than pushing too hard for change.

STRATEGY 2. BUILDING ON THE SCALING QUESTIONS

This strategy is *linked to the numerical assessment of confidence* described in Chapter 4. Once you are familiar with the process, it will be easy to adapt it to nonnumerical form, simply by asking questions. It is simply a way of opening the door to talk about strategies and targets. The patient, as you will see, does most of the thinking and talking, while your role is to ask questions and help with clarifying the stumbling blocks to change.

When you conducted your assessment of how confident the patient feels to make a particular change, he or she gave you a rating out of 10.

- You now have a platform for understanding exactly how the patient feels and what might lead to successful change. Keep the pace of the discussion slow, and adopt a curious attitude. Your hope is that the answers lie within the patient.

WHAT TO AVOID

With all your experience of helping people with behavior change, you often have lots of ideas how patients might go about it. Unfortunately, you do not know how they feel any of these ideas would fit into their own lives.

Practitioner: So you gave yourself a score of 3/10 for confidence to actually change your diet. What about cutting out those snacks between meals from now on? And wholemeal bread is much more filling, so if you made your sandwiches with that you wouldn't get so hungry mid-afternoon.

Patient: Yes but...!

It is more effective to elicit from patients what they think would work rather than bombarding them with suggestions.

- Ask either or both of the following questions and then follow them with other open questions or reflective listening statements. You will recognize these questions from the similar strategy for exploring importance.

Why so high?

Ask why the patient scored a given number and not a lower number: *You said that you were fairly confident about your ability to change* [behavior]. *Why have you scored 4 and not 1?* The answers could provide important clues for what might work in the future. For example: *I am at 4 and not 1 because I know that if the situation is right, if I can keep away from friends who push me in the wrong direction, I can succeed.* This will allow you to respond with observations like *So you've got the confidence to succeed if only you could organize your social life differently.* You can either pursue this in more detail or keep the focus broad to begin with by asking a question like *What other reasons do you have for giving yourself a score of 4 and not 1?*

How can you go higher?
You could also ask a quite different question: for example, *You gave yourself a score of 4. So you do have some confidence that you could succeed. How could you become more confident, so that your score goes up to 5 or 6?* or *What would help you to become more confident?* Note that one can ask about either *your score* or just *you.* The latter often feels better.

STRATEGY 3. BRAINSTORM SOLUTIONS
Some patients, in some situations, apparently want to be told what to do. Certainly, if someone has an acute life-threatening condition, he or she will probably take your advice. In most behavior change consultations, however, patients probably prefer greater autonomy of decision-making. If clinical judgment tells you that a patient really wants you to tell him or her what to do, then you should respond accordingly. However, most patients, we believe, will react against simple advice-giving.

How do you help with action plans without telling patients what to do? How do you avoid falling into an advice-giving trap: the patient wants to know what to do, you offer a constructive suggestion, and then the patient tells you why this will not work? The problem with simple advice-giving is that it can restrict patients' sense of autonomy (see Chapter 2). Faced with this threat, they react against your advice. More information about the concept of reactance can be found in Chapter 7. Another problem with advice-giving is that it usually takes the form of a single, simple piece of advice. Surely, if it was that simple, the patient would have tried it before. You do not know the patient's circumstances as well as he or she does!

The alternative to simple advice-giving is presented below in the form of a single strategy that can be learned quite quickly. In essence, rather than advising patients what to do, you encourage them to select targets and strategies for achieving them. Your expertise is used to enrich this process, not to overwhelm it. You construct a range of options with the patient and then encourage him or her to choose the most appropriate. You can suggest any number of options yourself, as long as you help the patient to choose the one that is most suitable. A good analogy is a menu. Menus offer suggestions and possibilities and may even offer explanations and the chef's recommendations, but the diner still gets to choose what to eat.

This maximizes patient participation, while allowing you to use your knowledge and expertise to enhance this process, not to replace it. This simple strategy is usually called *brainstorming*. However, the spirit of this process is just as important as matters of technique. This should be conveyed to the patient from the outset. For example, *There are usually not one but many possible courses of action. I can tell you about what's worked for other people but you will be the best judge of what works for you. Let's go through some of the options together.*

Identify a number of options. Encourage the patient to come up with as many as possible. Use your expertise in suggesting these options. Be careful about the patient becoming too passive. Try to avoid spending too much time evaluating the options. If the patient says, *Yes but, that won't work because…*, say something like *That's fine, let's not get too stuck on one idea, let's move on… what else might you do?*

When presenting an option, it can be useful to talk about what has worked for other patients. For example, *Some people in your situation have found it useful to…* Another useful question is *Are there any other ways that you know about that have worked for other people?* Your attitude should be one of neutrality about the possibilities. It is up to the patient to decide. This is the next step.

Let the patient select the most suitable option. Questions like *Which one suits you the best?* or *What makes the most sense to you?* will help the patient decide what to do. Your approach here is one of following patients' thought processes. Your task is to elicit and to understand how the patient really feels about what to do.

Convey optimism and willingness to reexamine. If the patient selects an option, let him or her know that if things do not work out, there will be other options that might work. It is a matter of working out what best suits the individual.

This strategy can be used to select a goal, strategy, or target (see Table 5.3).

STRATEGY 4. PAST EFFORTS: SUCCESSES AND FAILURES

Our expectations of ourselves are frequently related to past experiences. We can learn what we are good at and what we find most difficult by looking back at previous attempts to change. This can be a good way of learning; a slightly more sophisticated form of *trial and error*. However, sometimes people allow their confidence to be undermined by what they see as repeated failures.

Helping someone to see the past as a valuable piece of information, to help plan a more successful future, is a skill. Patients with low self-esteem may be particularly likely to recount stories of their "relapses" as evidence of their general worthlessness. *Policing the past*, as a colleague put it, can become a destructive part of clinic routine (N.C.H. Stott, personal communication). Here, the guilty patient feels obliged to explain failure to the well-meaning practitioner who routinely asks, *How have you been getting on?*, when the question was merely a device for starting the conversation about change.

A very common experience is for people to try and fail so many times that they become demoralized and lose their confidence. Very many people have repeatedly tried to lose weight or give up smoking. Affirm the person's hard work and persistence in trying more than once. Courage and perseverance are important. Patients can be encouraged to give themselves credit for applying these qualities to the issue under discussion. Encourage them, too, to see themselves as competent, determined people who are potentially able to make changes but have not yet hit on a successful plan for doing so.

Ask about the person's most successful attempt to date. What made it different from any other attempts? Are any of these differences things that could, deliberately, be built into a new plan? Solution-focused therapists emphasize the value of encouraging people to talk about their strengths rather than their difficulties and guiding conversations toward *solution talk* (Iveson and Ratner, 1990). They also look for exceptions, for even transient evidence that change is possible. If someone feels it would be impossible to go half an hour or more without a cigarette, check if he or she has ever succeeded, even if he or she was coerced rather than chose such an action. Perhaps the person went on holiday by air or found him- or herself in a social situation where escaping for a cigarette was impossible for an hour or so. If someone finds it difficult to imagine that he or she could refuse a drink offered by a friend, inquire if he or she has ever done so: for example, when driving or on medication. How offended was the friend? Can anything from that situation be transferred over to the present?

If patients acknowledge that they did change briefly but discount this, saying, *Yes but it was dreadfully hard — it nearly killed me,* they may be helped to reframe this as even more of a triumph; success in the face of almost overwhelming difficulty is worth more than success at an easy task: *Looking back on it now, you must be really impressed with yourself for coping with such a difficult situation!*

Keep the discussion of past experiences focused as much as possible on things that are and are seen by patients as being, within their control. If a previous attempt failed because of unforeseen circumstances, *I was doing well going to the gym twice a week but then my husband lost his job and we had to sell the car,* or *I was losing weight but then I became pregnant and things were very difficult with the pregnancy and I really couldn't keep going with the diet plan then,* acknowledge that there were real difficulties and move on to look at things that the patient could plan for and take control over another time.

WHAT TO AVOID

It is easy to be over-positive about people's previous successes or too dismissive of unsuccessful attempts when trying to build confidence. This may lead to resistance in the form of a restatement of the patient's lack of confidence and a "backing off" from the discussion. Look out for this and remain patient-centered.

STRATEGY 5. REASSESS CONFIDENCE

The assessment of importance and confidence was pinpointed in Chapter 4 as something from which to launch a conversation about behavior change. It can be useful on an ongoing basis in the consultation too, particularly when talking about confidence-building. When one starts to talk about specific strategies and targets for confidence-building, the levels of self-efficacy will vary across them. For example, someone wishing to drink less might be fairly confident about staying away from alcohol at home but less so about ordering soft drinks when out with friends.

To return to an assessment of levels of confidence can be very useful. This can be done formally, in numerical form, as described on p. 62, or it can be done informally, with a question like *We have talked about change X and change Y. Which of these do you feel more confident about succeeding with?* and later *Why do you feel this way?* The obvious guiding principle is to encourage change with which the patient is more likely to succeed.

REMINDERS ON ACTION PLANNING

Move from the general to the specific, not the other way around, i.e., from a goal, through strategies to targets.

- Help the patient set *small, achievable targets* if at all possible.
- Establish a *realistic time scale.* Changing habits and establishing a new lifestyle takes time and is a gradual process. Some people enjoy dramatic all-or-nothing-type changes and others cope better with gradual changes, one small step at a time. Choosing a day to begin the change can be important, as well as choosing the pace of change. A good time scale is one that is slow enough to be manageable but fast enough to show some results so as to keep up the patient's motivation. Useful questions include *One of the things you said you liked about drinking and would miss if you cut down was the socializing — I wonder how it will be if you start making changes right now? What are the next couple of weeks like socially?* or *You are a bit worried about your family's reaction if you start cooking the food with less fat; how could you go about it to avoid a mutiny?*
- Is the patient really ready? Sometimes patients are not as ready as you thought, perhaps still being in the contemplation stage. This can account for their apparent resistance to selecting an option. Reassess readiness to change at any point. Be open about this with patients.
- Failing to make action plans does not mean that the consultation has failed. Do not push the patient too far. Time spent with you can often lead to action being taken independently at a later point.
- Clarify how you will both monitor progress.
- If behavior change does not take place, it is more helpful for both of you to see the plan, rather than the patient, as inadequate.
- Acknowledge patients' concerns, do not ignore them. Ask about these, if possible without getting bogged down. Useful questions include *You did say that you really enjoy the feeling of relaxation that you get from smoking. How much do you think you'll miss that?*, or *Before we go on to plan how to change, are there any things that particularly concern you about the prospect of change? What went wrong last time you tried and how can we make it different this time?*

RESISTANCE AND BUILDING CONFIDENCE

If a patient resists your efforts to come up with a plan, consider which of the following might be the explanation:

- Are you focusing on building *confidence* when in fact the patient is not really convinced about the *importance* of the change under discussion? Consider a return to the task of exploring importance. You might even share this observation with the patient and allow him or her to be your guide.
- Are you overestimating the patient's level of confidence to succeed and unwittingly pushing him or her toward change? Back off! Consider reassessing confidence. Ask the patient how they really feel. Patients often simply cannot imagine coping without, say, a cigarette, a drink, or that special food in the refrigerator.
- Are you providing solutions rather than letting the patient discover them?
- Are you falling into the trap of talking about *single* solutions, when it is a little more complex for the patient?
- Are you looking at the *wrong* target or even the wrong strategy for achieving change (see Table 5.3)? Clarify this with the patient.

A CASE EXAMPLE OF BUILDING CONFIDENCE

Nurse: So you've tried to stop smoking lots of times before. How confident do you feel about having another go?

Patient: Not very.

Nurse: On a scale of 1–10, how confident do you feel? If 1 is "not at all confident" and 10 is "very confident"? [Uses scaling questions]

Patient: About 3 or 4.

Nurse: So, not very, but better than a 1 or a 2. Why is that? [Tries to elicit change talk]

Patient: Well, I tried cutting down gradually but that didn't work. I tried a "quit smoking" group where they made us stop completely on a particular day. I once had a go with nicotine gum. None of them worked in the long term but I did last 6 weeks once. That was with the quit group.

Nurse: What helped you to go so long that time? [Reviews the positives in the previous attempt]

Patient: I think it was better for me to stop completely. There was a nice woman in the group who I got on well with, and we encouraged each other. It went wrong when I started seeing a man who smoked heavily and I had one smoke one night and then just drifted back into it.

Nurse: So it sounds as if support from other people makes a big difference to you. It helps you to change [reviews positive experiences] and when you spend a lot of time with someone who doesn't support you, you are more likely to slip back. [Learns from previous failures] It also sounds as if a definite quit date helps you.

Patient: Yes. I'm not very good at doing things on my own. [Expresses low self-esteem in relation to behavior change, in general]

Nurse: There's nothing unusual about wanting support and that's why there are so many support groups set up. Shall we look at all the different ways you could get support this time if you decided to quit, and see how you feel about them? Because of all the experience you've had of trying to change in the past, you will be the best judge of what would work for you. [Goes on to explore options and exchanges information as part of this process]

The nurse encourages the patient to draw on his or her previous experiences, not to make him or her remember his or her failures but to identify how much he or she has learned about him- or herself and about stopping smoking. His or her confidence will be built by seeing that if he or she does decide to change, he or she can design his or her own action plan; incorporating the things he or she already knows can help him or her, and working out how to cope with things that he or she can predict will be difficult.

It is important that the nurse remembers throughout that although the patient has agreed that it is important to change, he or she has not yet decided to do so. Adding the phrase, *If you decided to quit,* into the discussion about action plans avoids raising the resistance that might have been elicited by an implied assumption that the patient will change.

OVERLAPPING OF IMPORTANCE AND CONFIDENCE

The possibility of importance and confidence issues being interconnected was discussed briefly in Chapter 4. In earlier stages of readiness, there is often a clear distinction between them; importance is usually low and is probably the dimension on which you need to focus. In later stages of readiness, however, the perceived benefits and costs of change tend to hinge on confidence issues. For example, many overweight patients have no doubt about the value of change, but because they have low levels of confidence, the perceived value of change is depressed accordingly. One of the obstacles they anticipate which devalues change is an inability to control their eating in different situations.

Thus, when working with strategies applicable to fairly high levels of importance, the distinction between importance and confidence can become blurred, not with every patient but certainly with some of them. Use of strategies like exploring concerns or a hypothetical look over the fence can thus involve discussion of confidence issues as well. Learning to move between these two dimensions in the melting pot of later stages of readiness is certainly a challenge. If you get confused, ask the patient where the conversation should go next, as your task is not to solve problems but to encourage patients to do this themselves.

BOX 5.1 USEFUL QUESTIONS
Explore importance
1. What would have to happen for it to become much more important for you to change?
2. What would have to happen before you seriously considered changing?
3. Why have you given yourself such a high score on importance?
4. What would need to happen for your importance score to move up from X to Y?
5. What stops you moving up from X to Y?
6. What are the good things about... [current behavior]? What are some of the less good things about... [current behavior]? [Alternative: things you like and dislike...]
7. What concerns do you have about... [current behavior]?
8. If you were to change, what would it be like?
9. Where does this leave you now? [When you want to ask about change in a neutral way]

Build confidence
1. What would make you more confident about making these changes?
2. Why have you given yourself such a high score on confidence?
3. How could you move up higher, so that your score goes from X to Y?
4. How can I help you succeed?
5. Is there anything you found helpful in any previous attempts to change?
6. What have you learned from the way things went wrong last time you tried?
7. If you were to decide to change, what might your options be? Are there any ways you know about that have worked for other people?
8. What are some of the practical things you would need to do to achieve this goal? Do any of them sound achievable?
9. Is there anything you can think of that would help you feel more confident?

CONCLUSION

The skill required when talking to patients about the *why*, *how*, *what*, and *when* of behavior change is not a matter of applying strategies *to* them but of structuring a conversation in a useful way which encourages the patient to take as much of the lead as possible. Above all, it is about constructive listening and joint decision-making. The strategies described in this chapter are merely guides to structuring this kind of consultation.

KEY POINTS
- There is more than one right way to explore importance.
- There is more than one right way to build confidence.
- Stay with patients in terms of their readiness to change. Only move on to action planning when you receive a message that the patient feels ready to do so.

REFERENCES

Arkowitz, H., Westra, H.A., Miller, W.R., Rollnick, S., 2008. Motivational Interviewing in the Treatment of Psychological Problems. Guilford Press, New York.

Bandura, A., 1977. Towards a unifying theory of behavior change. Psychological Review 84, 191–215.

de Shazer, S., Berg, I., Lipchick, E., et al., 1986. Brief therapy: a focused solution development. Family Process 25, 207–222.

Egan, G., 1994. The Skilled Helper: A Problem Management Approach to Helping. Brooks/Cole, Pacific Grove.

Iveson, G., Ratner, H., 1990. Problem to Solution. Brief Therapy Press, London.

Miller, W.R., 1983. Motivational interviewing with problem drinkers. Behavioral Psychotherapy 1, 147–172.

Miller, W.R., Rollnick, S., 2012. Motivational Interviewing: Helping People Change, third ed. Guilford Press, New York.

Orford, J., 2001. Excessive Appetites: A Psychological View of Addictions, second ed. Wiley, Chichester.

Rollnick, S., Heather, N., Bell, A., 1992. Negotiating behavior change in medical settings: the development of brief motivational interviewing. Journal of Mental Health 1, 25–37.

Rollnick, S., Butler, C.C., Stott, N., 1997. Helping smokers make decisions: the enhancement of brief intervention for general medical practice. Patient Education and Counseling 31, 191–203.

Exchanging information

CHAPTER OUTLINE

INTRODUCTION

There are two tasks that a practitioner might need to perform at various stages throughout a consultation: exchanging information with the patient and responding constructively to resistance. This chapter describes the first.

An overweight young woman is referred "for dietary and fitness advice." She sits down by your desk a little apprehensive and expectant. The overall task, as you both know, is to set her on the path to successful weight loss. You need to know some key things about her before you can imagine what might work for her. She is expecting you to give her information about diets and exercise. You expect that she has probably dieted before and has some knowledge and ideas about how to do it. You need to know how much she already knows and how accurate her existing information is.

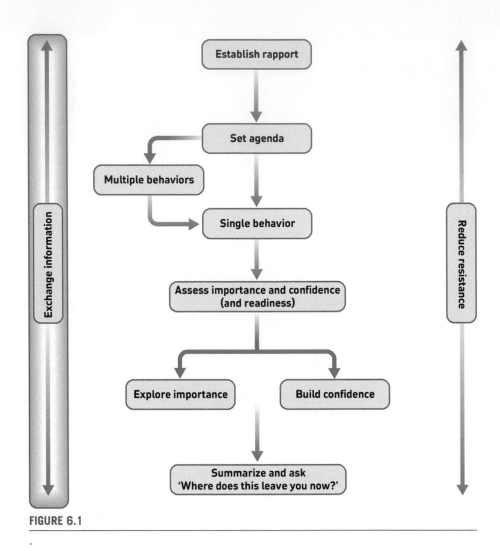

FIGURE 6.1

.

You want her to leave the consultation with all the accurate information she needs to make a success of a weight loss program.

A middle-aged man has been diagnosed with liver disease. You need to discuss with him the importance of stopping drinking alcohol. You do not know whether he already realizes that he needs to think about his drinking. You do not know what part alcohol plays in his life and how much he would mind giving it up. You know a lot about strategies for giving up drinking and places he could get support, and you would like to give him as much of this information as possible.

A large part of the practitioner's role is giving information to the patient. A large part of the patient's role is giving information to the practitioner.

Done badly, this task will make the patient a passive recipient of expert knowledge, disconnected from his or her context and concerns. Done well, it is a vehicle

> **BOX 6.1 USEFUL QUESTIONS**
> **Exchange information**
> 1. Would you like to know more about...?
> 2. How much do you already know about?
> 3. The test result is... X, what do you make of this?
> 4. What happens to some people is... and... What about you?
> 5. How do you see the connection between X and Y?
> 6. Now that I have given you this information, how does it apply to you?
> 7. Take me through a typical day in your life, and tell me where your [behavior] fits in? ...So, on Monday, you woke up, how were you feeling? ...Then what did you do? ...You're going a bit fast for me! Can I take you back to when you left the house on Monday morning... What happened then, and how did you feel?

for true understanding and, it appears, a better outcome. For the practitioner, information exchange will be linked to specific medical or behavioral matters. For the patient, it often also includes broader personal concerns. To deal with the former at the expense of the latter can be a serious mistake. Improving various aspects of the information exchange process can enhance the congruence between patient and practitioner and encourage the patient to think positively about change. This is not just a "technical matter" or an exercise in the exchange of facts but something that involves the use of skillful listening, careful questioning, and well-timed intervention. There are few parts of the consultation that do not involve the eliciting or providing of information.

Studies of communication reveal that the way in which practitioners exchange information can be strikingly one-sided and, at times, insensitive. For example, one study found that practitioners interrupted patients an average of 18 s into their initial description of the problem; in another study, patients and practitioners did not agree on the main presenting problem in 50% of outpatient consultations (Starfield et al., 1981).

Given its obvious importance, it is something of a surprise to notice that information exchange is seldom taught as a specific topic in its own right. It is difficult to find clear and teachable strategies that help practitioners to carry out this task. Rather, they are left to find their own ways of doing this. The purpose of this chapter is to bring together what we understand as the most effective and satisfying way to exchange information, in a form that can be learned and practiced and readily integrated into day-to-day consultations. This not only is relevant to behavior change conversations but also applies to other kinds of consultations, such as when breaking bad news, talking about diagnoses, and so on.

The lack of progress in developing such methods is not just a practical problem but also a conceptual one. Information exchange has been too readily viewed as a one-sided process, hence the emphasis in both research and practice on either *assessment* (getting information *from* the patient) or *feedback* (giving information *to* the patient), both of which are activities derived mainly from the agenda of the practitioner. The education of medical and other students is usually guided by this kind of one-sided approach. Rees and Williams (2009) reviewed the patient–practitioner encounter with adults living in the community with physical chronic illness and found that "for effective patient-centeredness to be established patients should be able to discuss their own ideas about self-care actions, including lifestyle management in an unhurried fashion and with a practitioner who has the time and who is willing to listen."

As the strategies described below will reveal, the conceptual framework being used is explicitly two sided, where the practitioner also encourages the patient to drive the discussion at certain points in the exchange process. Thus, the patient will not only be assessed and receive feedback but will also express his or her information needs and be encouraged to arrive at a personal interpretation of the information received.

Conceived thus, information exchange is a skillful task which will benefit from further development work and careful attention to the process of how best to improve practice. The practical strategies below come from two sources: first, the study of communication and the patient-centered method, and second, motivational interviewing.

THE PATIENT-CENTERED METHOD AND WHAT HAPPENS IF WE CHANGE PATIENTS' BEHAVIOR IN CONSULTATIONS

Research on communication, going back many years, reveals, as one might expect, that practitioners vary considerably in how they exchange information and that outcome can be improved if information is clear and simple and if practitioners negotiate and agree on treatment goals in a cooperative manner (Becker, 1985). Although these findings are obviously useful, much of the research on compliance is based on the notion that behavior change is best "induced" by the expert-driven delivery of clear information, a view we explicitly reject (see Butler et al., 1996).

Of more direct relevance, has been the work on patient empowerment and the patient-centered method carried out by a number of North American research teams. Not all of this research focuses on information exchange, although a number of studies, reviewed by Stewart (1995), have looked explicitly at the process of history-taking. Four correlational studies, all of them in outpatient settings, reveal that during history-taking, activities like a full discussion of the problem, the asking of questions by the patient, providing information, and giving emotional support are all associated with better outcomes, such as the resolution of headaches and numerous other physical symptoms. Two randomized controlled trials found that practitioner training in history-taking improved levels of psychological distress in patients, and another two studies found that brief patient education (20 min) in how to ask questions not only improved participation but also led to improved physical health such as control of blood pressure and blood glucose levels.

Of course, information exchange does not only occur during history-taking. A number of other studies of patient empowerment have involved the training of patients to be more assertive in other phases of the consultation. Thus, Innui et al. (1976)

found that giving patients greater control over what is talked about and encouraging them to seek personally relevant information can improve outcomes like control of blood pressure. Greenfield et al. (1988) demonstrated that people with diabetes who were trained to be more involved in the consultation had better health outcomes than those who were not trained. Similarly, patients seen by health educators and coached to ask questions made better use of appointments over the following months (Roter, 1977). Therefore, this approach is by no means new, conceptually. The challenge has been to translate research findings into better practice across the clinical environment.

Finally, it is worth taking note of Silverman's (1997) observation of a feature of advice-giving, which avoids being too personal and eliciting resistance: If the advice is couched in terms of general information, i.e., in a broader, more neutral context, patients seem more likely to respond favorably.

In summary, there is clear evidence that if patients are more assertive during information exchange, outcomes can be improved. There is much less evidence that practitioners can be trained to improve their skills. There are clear correlations between elements of good-quality information exchange and patient outcome.

MOTIVATIONAL INTERVIEWING

A second source of innovation comes from the early work of William R. Miller on motivational interviewing in the addictions field. He found a way of training counselors to encourage curiosity, question-asking and personal reflection among clients about the meaning of information provided to them. This process, it turns out, can have a powerful effect on people's decision-making. It appears that this is a matter not just of presenting appropriate information clearly to people but of distinguishing between "facts" and their interpretation. In these drinkers' check-up studies (see Miller and Sovereign, 1989), the counselor provided the facts in a nonjudgmental, neutral manner, and then encouraged the patient, through the use of simple open questions, to arrive at a personal interpretation of them. More detail about this process can be found in Miller et al. (1988). The ideal outcome would be for the patient to say or think, *I see, I never thought about it like this before, I wonder if this means that…* Strategy 1, outlined below, is based on this aspect of motivational interviewing. It was refined further in the development of brief motivational interviewing (Rollnick et al., 1992), where a clearly defined and documented information exchange strategy was taught to a group of general health-care workers doing health promotion work with heavy drinkers in a general hospital (Heather et al., 1996). Rollnick et al. (2008) devote a whole chapter to the skills of informing in the context of motivational interviewing in a health-care setting, and note that, "a relationship, even if it lasts no more than a few minutes, lies at the heart of informing" (p. 88).

What emerges from these developments is a view of information exchange as part of a delicately balanced conversation. It does not need to be a sterile, expert-driven activity. From a conceptual viewpoint, we do not adhere to the view of information exchange as a practitioner-driven process either of eliciting facts from patients (assessment) or of providing them with information (feedback). In both such activities, the patient will be driven along by the agenda of the practitioner, who will do most of the talking. Instead, we view the process in terms of the following circular *elicit—provide—elicit* process described below (Strategy 1).

What should happen if the practitioner has a very genuine desire to gather specific information from a patient close to the beginning of a consultation? How can one avoid firing, say, 20 closed questions at the patient? It is not that this kind of assessment has no place in a consultation. It can be useful, particularly when a reasonable rapport has been established, and it is done in a clear and logical manner. However, the interest here has been in finding a way of helping practitioners to gather information that was based more on a conversation, in a more patient-centered way. What emerged was the *Typical Day strategy* mentioned in Chapter 3 and described in detail below (Strategy 2), in which the patient is simply encouraged to tell a story about a typical day. It is a delight to see the way in which facts come tumbling out in this kind of account. It does take up to 6—10 min to use and might therefore be beyond the scope of many consultations. If time is available, however, the use of this strategy is recommended as a viable alternative to asking the patient a large number of direct questions at the beginning of a consultation. Crucially, it helps to cement the rapport between the parties.

In summary, information exchange is an art as much as a technique or procedure. It is as much about maintaining rapport and having a conversation, as it is about the exchange of facts. The two strategies outlined below are designed to help practitioners to achieve these goals.

FEARFUL INFORMATION: WHO WANTS IT?

There is no shortage of fearful information in health-care consultations, and usually it is the practitioner who decides that it will do the patient good to hear about it. Unfortunately, being concerned about risks and negative outcomes is not always a precipitant of change. We can all tell stories of patients who *increase* their risky behavior in the face of frightening information or experiences. Research in health psychology seems to bear this out (Schwarzer and Fuchs, 1996). There are many other more positive motives for change, often little to do with health as such. If the patient asks about health risks and negative consequences, then of course it is appropriate to provide this. It is also appropriate to offer information if you believe the patient does not already have it: for example, *We know a bit more than we used to about how being overweight can affect the medical condition you have. Would you be interested in my updating you on that?* However, we should probably be careful of making a habit of providing frightening stories or facts. The best habit is probably to routinely ask patients what they would like to know.

What about people getting all their information from the Internet?

Because this book was first written, a big change has occurred. When people get sick now the first thing many of us do is "google" it and look it up on our search engine. It is also what we do when we get home from a consultation; look it up and check what the clinician said and crossmatch with our symptoms. Then again we might check out chat rooms etc. for ideas on complementary therapies that might have been overlooked by the practitioner but which might bring relief and next time we attend the clinic go armed with a list of treatments we have read and want to try.

This drives clinicians crazy as they feel they now have to deal with people who are unnecessarily terrified by what they have read or misread or who are unrealistically hopeful of a magic cure. Patients do not seem to trust their health-care teams any more, and it feels as if patient empowerment seems to lead to practitioner loss of power.

Grünloh et al. (2018) explore this in a qualitative study with 12 physicians and found that although they all supported patient empowerment in theory, their daily practice did not support this. They suggest that interactions need to be seen more as "sense-making and learning activities" for patients to help them to make sense of what they have read and conflicting advice they may have encountered.

So the practitioner's role may be evolving from having a major role in informing patients to helping them to process all the information they have themselves amassed and working out the implications for their own condition and circumstances.

TWO STRATEGIES FOR EXCHANGING INFORMATION
STRATEGY 1. ELICIT—PROVIDE—ELICIT (GENERAL INFORMATION EXCHANGE)

This strategy is mainly for situations where you are thinking of giving the patient information. First, patients are encouraged to describe their behavior, ask questions, indicate what they would most like to know, or disclose what they do and do not know about a particular topic (*elicit*). Unlike the more traditional approach, the practitioner is encouraged to adopt a curious and eliciting interviewing style during this phase, and the patient will do most of the talking. This is what is commonly called *assessment*. Second, the practitioner is active in conveying clear, nonjudgmental information (*provide*) which, crucially, in the third phase, the patient is given an opportunity to absorb and reflect on (*elicit*). We have distinguished between these three phases to develop teachable strategies. In reality, of course, they are usually interlinked and might not follow a clear and logical sequence. This is not a problem. It is the spirit of information exchange that is most important. Consider the following sequences:

ELICIT readiness and interest
Ask the patient if he or she would like information, and about what? For example, *Would you like to know more about...?* or *How much do you know about...?* [Then later] *Would you like to know how...?* Do not rush this process. Take your time to

understand what information, if any, the patient requires. If you get the feeling that the patient does not really want any information, back off and withdraw. In fact, do not appear too enthusiastic or evangelical about the whole process! If they say they do not want information and you go on and give it anyway, they are unlikely to be receptive at this time.

PROVIDE information neutrally

Offer objective facts, and try to avoid using the term *you*. One way of achieving this is to refer to other people and what happens to them. This is less threatening to the receiver and is thus more likely to be heard accurately. This knowledge about other patients' experiences is also the true source of your expertise. For example, *What happens to some people is that… Other people find that…*

ELICIT the patient's interpretation and follow it

Now is the time to use the word *you*! The aim is to encourage the patient to make sense of the meaning of the information. For example, *What do you make of this? I wonder how you have been affected by…? How does this fit in with how you see things?* Follow the patient's reaction for as long as you are able. This process of integrating information is what will help build motivation to change. It is the most important part of this process and the part most often forgotten. Practitioners sometimes think it is their job to give information. It might be more accurate to say that the job is to help patients to hear and make sense and use of information.

The following principles are important throughout:

- Does the patient want or need information? About what? How much does he or she already know? There is no point in providing irrelevant information or that which the patient does not want to receive. The best time to provide information is when the patient asks for it.
- Make a distinction, if at all possible, between factual information and the personal interpretation of it. You present the information and encourage the patient to interpret its meaning.
- Use language you think the patient understands.
- When presenting information, present it in a neutral tone of voice and avoid too much use of the word *you*.
- Keep the pacing congruent with the patient's uptake of the information; pause regularly to observe uptake and comprehension.
- Paint a general picture first, and then move into specifics as the patient directs you. Filling in too much detail can confuse the patient.

WHAT TO AVOID

Too easily, people interpret being given information as being told what to do. Their response then may well be one of reactance rather than curiosity and interest. Our aim is to make it clear that we are sharing our knowledge of the facts so that *they* can make a decision about what to do.

Taking information home

The principles described above also apply to information offered for taking home. Avoid *distributing* information to patients. Assess their readiness to receive it first, and explain where in the literature or other media they might locate the information most relevant to them. Invite them to return for further discussion, and when you do see them again, ask how it went with looking at it and whether there is anything in it they want to discuss.

STRATEGY 2. A TYPICAL DAY (GATHERING INFORMATION)

This strategy is mainly for situations where your focus is on gathering information from the patient, rather than imparting it to them. It emerged in the development of brief motivational interviewing (see Rollnick et al., 1992), in the search for a way of conducting assessment in the form of a conversation led by the patient. The strategy fits in well with this approach and is easily learned. It provides the practitioner with a profusion of hard facts (usually the object of formal assessment) and also gives a clear idea about the relevant personal context of health behavior. Its usefulness extends beyond information exchange. It is ideal for establishing rapport. If focused on a particular behavior and its place in the person's life, it can also help to establish readiness to change.

This strategy involves simply asking the patient to take you through a typical day in his or her life. It is described here with reference to a particular behavior or problem, although this is obviously not essential. Having agreed to talk about a particular behavior or problem (e.g., diabetes), you can launch straight into this strategy. It can take as little as 3–5 min to use, although the ideal time is about 6–8 min; too much longer and it can become tiresome for both parties. Of course, the strategy does not have to focus on a typical *day*. One can ask about a typical drinking or eating binge, a typical afternoon, or whatever.

The examination of a typical day, as opposed to, for example, a really difficult day or a particularly good day, is somewhat arbitrary. One could use one of the latter approaches, but our preference is for a focus on the normal, not the abnormal, as a device for establishing rapport and understanding the general context. Quite often, people tell you about the abnormal as part of this process. It is a conversation, not an investigation.

The spirit of this strategy is the most important; it is like asking the patient to paint a picture. Your role is simply to try to understand what is being painted. You might ask for a bit more detail here or there, but your task is simply to understand. The interviewing style is curious rather than interrogative. This strategy is easy to practice with patients. It is unlikely to cause discomfort. In broad outline, it takes the following forms.

Introduce the task carefully

Sit back and relax! Ask the patient a question like *Can you take me through a typical day in your life, so that I can understand in more detail what happens?* [Then, if you are talking about a particular behavior] *Then you can also tell me where your* [eating/ smoking/drinking/etc.] *fits in. Can you think of a recent typical day? Take me through this day from beginning to end. You got up…*

Follow the story

- Allow the patient to paint a picture with as little interruption as possible. Listen carefully. Simple open questions are usually all you need; for example, *What happened then? How did you feel? What exactly made you feel that way?*
- Avoid imposing any of your hypotheses, ideas, or interesting questions on the story you are being told. Hold them back for a later time. This is the biggest mistake made when first using this strategy. Do not investigate problems!
- Watch the pacing. If it is a bit slow, speed things up: *Can you take us forward a bit more quickly? What happened when…?* If it is a bit too fast, slow things down: *Hold on! You are going too fast. Take me back to… What happened…?*
- If you are uncertain about details and you are happy that you are being curious rather than investigative, then ask the patient to fill them in for you.
- You know you have got it right when you are doing 10%–15% of the talking, the patient seems engaged in the process, and lots of interesting information about the person is emerging.

Review and summarize

Sometimes this is unnecessary, and you can move on to another topic. If you do pause to take stock, a useful question is *Is there anything else at all about this picture you have painted that you would like to tell me?* This is also a good opportunity to be honest with the patient about your reaction and to provide affirmation wherever you can. Having listened so carefully to the patient, you will now be able to change the topic quite easily. Often this leads into the general information exchange strategy described above, introduced, for example, by, *Is there anything about… that you would like to know?*

A CASE EXAMPLE OF EXCHANGING INFORMATION

Patient: I do realize I ought to be more active but I don't really know where to start.
Practitioner: What do you know about how much exercise is recommended to keep the body healthy?
Patient: Not much really. In the old days doctors told our parents to touch their toes every day and now people go to gyms and so on.
Practitioner: Would you be interested in me taking a moment to tell you what we medical folks recommend?
Patient: Yes, please.

Practitioner: The general guideline is that people take a minimum of 30 min, 5 days a week, to do something active that leaves them warm and slightly out of breath. Some people do this through formal "exercise," and others build it into their life by walking or cycling to work, gardening etc.

Patient: So I don't need to go to the gym or buy a dance class DVD? I can do more everyday stuff?

Practitioner: It sounds as if you think there are ways you could get that 30 min of doing something strenuous built into your daily routine.

Patient: Well, I was just thinking about walking to work. It would take about 25 min, I should think, and by the time I've got stuck in rush-hour traffic and found somewhere to park, it takes me nearly that long to drive. I wouldn't want to do it on wet days though. What else could I do? Does the 30 min need to be all in one go?

Practitioner: No, we used to think so but they've now found people can add together little bits of exercise such as climbing the stairs. Does that give you any more ideas?

Patient: It is certainly starting to sound more possible.

Practitioner: Would you like to tell me about a typical day for you at the moment and how physical activity fits in at the moment? You said you drive to work. How active are you in your job once you get there?

HOW DOES INFORMATION RELATE TO IMPORTANCE AND CONFIDENCE?

When we look at the times when we feel driven to give information, it is usually either in the hope of enhancing patients' perception of the importance of change or with the expectation that they will feel more confident about achieving it once they hear what we have to say.

For example, a smoking cessation advisor may want to tell a pregnant smoker about the domiciliary smoking cessation counseling offered by a specialist midwife. She hopes that the woman will feel more confident about quitting once she knows that the support will come to her rather than her having to arrange childcare for her older child and struggle into town to a group.

Another example might be a doctor treating a heavy drinker with high blood pressure. The doctor wants to tell him about the effect that alcohol has on blood pressure because he would then see how it would help him to drink less. He might see changing his drinking as more important once he sees it is linked to a specific condition that is troubling him.

So, you might exchange information along the way while exploring importance or building confidence and then move back into whatever strategies you were using, seeing if that information has changed the *pros* and *cons* at all, or if it has changed the position on one of the scaling dimensions.

HOW IS INFORMATION EXCHANGE DIFFERENT FROM GIVING ADVICE?

The word "advice" is loosely used but usually entails some overt or covert offering of an opinion based on the advice-giver's interpretation of the facts. Information is the factual foundation on which good advice is built. We know for a fact that smoking is bad for health, and this may lead to advising a smoker to quit. In this patient-centered approach, the way forward is to give information but not to tell the patient what they should do with that information. If we give advice, we are saying what we think someone else should do, and this does not fit with the spirit of this way of working. Information, on the other hand, might cover

- reasons why many people choose to change
- results of medical tests and scans that throw light on the state of the patient's health
- ways that others have found helpful in changing
- services and support available to those who want to change

However, the decision about what is best for the patient is left for the patient to decide. This is a subtle difference in some ways but, in our experience, really makes a difference to the *feel* of the consultation and the level of resistance shown by patients. If a patient asks *What would you advise me to do?,* an alternative to giving advice, as such, is to say in an information-giving way, *I've seen people handle this in different ways… X works for some people and Y for others.* And then ask, *Could one of those ideas be adapted to work for you, do you think?* If someone really does want advice, *What do you think I should do?,* then you might, of course, choose to give it, and as it was solicited rather than imposed, the patient might even take it!

KEY POINTS

- Giving neutral information can be different from giving advice.
- You and the patient are a team. You know the scientific facts and have experience of what has helped other patients. The patient knows about his or her own life and body. If you collaborate, you have the complete picture.

REFERENCES

Becker, M.H., 1985. Patient adherence to prescribed therapies. Medical Care 23, 539–555.

Butler, C.C., Rollnick, S., Stott, N.C.H., 1996. The practitioner, the patient and resistance to change: recent ideas on compliance. Canadian Medical Association Journal 154, 1357–1362.

Greenfield, S., Kaplan, S.H., Ware, J.E., Yano, E.M., Frank, H.J., 1988. Patients' participation in medical care: effects on blood sugar control and quality of life in diabetes. Journal of General Internal Medicine 3, 448–457.

Grünloh, C., Myreteg, G., Cajander, A., Rexhepi, H., January 15, 2018. Why do they need to check me?' Patient participation through e-health and the doctor-patient relationship: qualitative study. Journal of Medical Internet Research 20 (1).

Heather, N., Rollnick, S., Bell, A., Richmond, R., 1996. Effects of brief counselling among male heavy drinkers identified on general hospital wards. Drug and Alcohol Review 15, 29–38.

Innui, T.S., Yourtree, E.L., Williamson, J., 1976. Improved outcomes in hypertension after physician tutorials. Internal Medicine 84, 646–651.

Miller, W., Sovereign, R.G., Krege, B., 1988. Motivational interviewing with problem drinkers: II. The drinker's check-up as a preventative intervention. Behavioral Psychotherapy 16, 251–268.

Miller, W.R., Sovereign, R.G., 1989. The check-up: a model for early intervention in addictive behaviors. In: Loberg, T., Miller, W.R., Nathan, P.E., Marlatt, G.A. (Eds.), Addictive Behaviors: Prevention and Early Intervention. Swets & Zeitlinger, Amsterdam.

Rees, S., Williams, A., 2009. Promoting and supporting self-management for adults living in the community with physical chronic illness: a systematic review of the effectiveness and meaningfulness of the patient-practitioner encounter. JBI Library of Systematic Reviews 7 (13), 492–582.

Rollnick, S., Heather, N., Bell, A., 1992. Negotiating behavior change in medical settings: the development of brief motivational interviewing. Journal of Mental Health 1, 25–37.

Rollnick, S., Miller, W.R., Butler, C., 2008. Motivational Interviewing in Health Care: Helping Patients Change Behavior. Guilford Press, New York.

Roter, D.L., 1977. Patient participation in the patient provider interaction: the effects of question asking on the quality of interaction, satisfaction, compliance. Health Education Monograph 5, 281–315.

Schwarzer, R., Fuchs, R., 1996. Self-efficacy and health behaviors. In: Conner, M., Norman, P. (Eds.), Predicting Health Behavior: Research and Practice with Social Cognition Models. Open University Press, Buckingham.

Silverman, D., 1997. Discourses in Counselling: HIV Counselling as Social Interaction. Sage, London.

Starfield, B., Wray, C., Hess, K., Gross, R., Birk, P.S., D'Lugoff, B.C., 1981. The influence of patient–practitioner agreement on outcome of care. American Journal of Public Health 71, 127–131.

Stewart, M., 1995. Effective physician–patient communication and health outcomes: a review. Canadian Medical Association Journal 152, 1423–1433.

Reducing resistance

CHAPTER OUTLINE

INTRODUCTION

Mrs. Green's weight is a real problem. She says she would love to be slim. She is unresponsive, however, to any of your suggestions about healthy eating or physical activity. She does not accept that her weight is connected to her behavior in these areas; she says she hardly eats a thing and is always rushing around burning up energy. She is convinced the problem is "glandular" or genetic in some way. You don't know how to help when she won't accept your suggestions.

    Her husband, on the other hand, agrees with you that it would be good for him to be more active. However, for every good idea you have, he has a reason why he cannot do it. He hates ball games, he can't afford to join a gym, walking to and from work is too dangerous in his neighborhood with the late shifts he does, and the pool isn't open at hours that suit him.

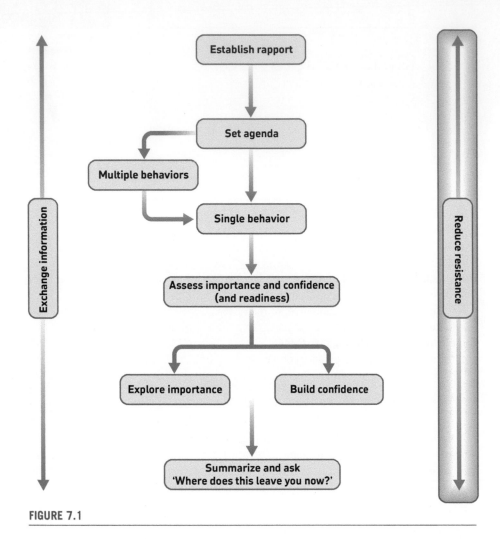

FIGURE 7.1

Some patients seem to resist your best efforts to help them. You think you are making good progress and then it all gets difficult again.

The discussion that follows leans unashamedly on motivational interviewing, with the goal of identifying some of the most useful ideas that can be applied to brief consultations. The three practical strategies that follow are simply examples of the ways in which practitioners can respond to resistance. It is an area with rich potential for further development and research. This chapter focuses on generally applicable strategies. Later, in Chapter 9, we look at a range of problem consultations that could clearly benefit from further development work; for example, in talk about chronic pain or chronic fatigue syndrome where the levels of resistance can be very high. Other useful ideas can be found in the work of Egan (1994), who captures much of what is said in this chapter by noting, "Effective helpers neither court reluctance or resistance nor are surprised by it" (p. 151).

WHAT IS RESISTANCE?

It is difficult to imagine a behavior change consultation that is not typically visited by resistance. It arises when there is tension or disagreement about behavior change. As this can arise at any point in the consultation, it requires continual watchfulness. Its equivalent in dancing is the paying of attention to keeping yourself and your partner from stepping on each other's toes. Maintaining a lightness of touch is essential.

Miller and Rollnick in 2012 look in detail at different aspects of client speech against change and distinguish between discord and sustain talk. Discord is when the client argues, challenges, or perhaps withdraws somehow as a response to a breakdown in the empathic therapeutic relationship. Typically they might, for example, feel judged and respond by defending themselves. They might feel misunderstood and challenge the practitioner's credentials, "*Who are you to tell me…, what do you know about…?*" Sustain talk, on the other hand, is a genuine explanation to the practitioner of reasons why it might be undesirable or too difficult to change, "*you see the problem is….I don't see how that would work for me….*" It is a verbalization of one side of the ambivalence. There is a third concept that is useful here; the psychology of reactance. This was first described in 1966 by Brehm and reviewed by Miron and Brehm 40 years later (2006). There is a large literature on this strong urge to retain a freedom, which occurs after it has been lost or threatened. Reactance is what leads us to so often resisting the social influence of others.

A common sequence is when the practitioner makes lots of helpful suggestions to the patient, *Why don't you…* and the patient responds to each with, *Yes, but…* Practitioners then think they have not yet come up with a helpful enough idea and generate more suggestions, only to be met with more explanations of why each would not work.

In many health-care consultations, there appears to be less outright conflict than in other settings, perhaps because time is shorter and patients do not have such a history of conflict with those caring for them. Patients are also sometimes in awe of doctors in particular and do not feel assertive enough to argue outright, so the resistance is hidden behind unenthusiastic apparent compliance. Practitioners, for their part, sometimes tread a skillful path to avoid conflict (Butler et al., 1998). Certainly, practitioners know that one way to avoid resistance is not to raise the subject of behavior change in the first place. This delicate management of resistance is well illustrated in the account of Silverman (1997), who describes quiet reluctance (e.g., *Uhmm ok….*) from patients more commonly than outright rejection. The need to "save face" by both parties is thought to be one explanation for this (Silverman, 1997). In some recordings of consultations about coughs, colds, and sore throats, where discomfort for doctors about whether or not to prescribe antibiotics is well documented in the literature by Bradley (1992), who found very little resistance and reached the conclusion that both parties conduct a delicate dance around the subject of antibiotics. Patients are seldom asked outright whether they want this medication, and doctors often avoid mentioning the word. However, both parties know it is a central issue. In other words, the subject of resistance is not new to health-care practitioners and patients; many are artful managers of tension in talk about change! Here, for simplicity, the term "resistance" is used to include all expressions of reluctance, resistance, and talk against change as the strategies for avoiding or managing them are similar.

WHAT CAUSES RESISTANCE?

Resistance can arise when the patient brings conflict into the consulting room, when the practitioner elicits it, or as a result of a combination of the two.

The patient can be in a state of internal conflict about change in which different voices in the mind are pressing for different outcomes: *I want to but it's so difficult…; I may as well just carry on…; If I could only try one more time…* On the one hand, they want to change, and on the other hand, they want to hold back from doing so. The resistance side of the argument can arise from: *It's too difficult; The whole thing* (condition) *is out of my control; There's a lot I like about the way things are now; I don't like anyone telling me what to do.*

When the patient is thinking privately about this, both sides of the argument are considered. They swing between *It would be good to…* and *I really don't want to.* When they are in conversation with someone else, if the other person (e.g., the practitioner) takes one side of the argument, *It would really help you if you could change…,* the patient will naturally respond with the opposing view, *But it's not that easy.* The same argument that was going on within the patient gets played out between the two of them, and practitioners frequently feel that they are fighting losing battles trying to help people who are just being resistant.

If the person is in conflict with others as well, it can be even more pronounced: *She always nags me about my diet, but she's the one who makes the food in the first place. What does she expect?* And sometimes the person might not be in a state of conflict but one of learned helplessness about lifestyle change. For example, some patients with chronic conditions like diabetes develop an almost habitual feeling of reluctance to change their lifestyles, and the routine check-up is characterized by reluctance from the patient and frustration for the practitioner. The more someone feels obliged to attend an appointment, the more likely it is that resistance will dog the consultation from the start.

Whatever the personal source of resistance for patients, they will be particularly sensitive to the way in which they are spoken. Problems usually arise in the consultation when, wittingly or unwittingly, the practitioner, wanting to encourage change, elicits from the patient a voice for no change: *Have you thought about controlling your diet?* The bar is raised, and the stage is set for the emergence of resistance: *Yes, but…*

In some circumstances, resistance can arise in the complete absence of conflict in the patient, when it is only the practitioner who is concerned about change. For example, a heavy drinker with no associated medical problems and who has never thought about alcohol use as a problem is at the receiving end of a health promotion effort intended to minimize future complications. If the practitioner implies that alcohol use is a problem, resistance is a predictable outcome. More common, probably, is where the origin of resistance is not as extreme as in this example, and there is an interaction between the conflict experienced by the patient and the motives and consulting behavior of the practitioner. Thus, whatever its origins, resistance cannot be defined outside of this interpersonal context. The practitioner has the potential to lower or raise the level of resistance.

DEALING WITH RESISTANCE

It is unrealistic to view resistance as a sign of failure in the consultation, as something that is abnormal and that should be eliminated from the discussion at all costs. Some therapists even say that with good rapport, resistance provides the kind of energy that generates change. However, in most time-limited health-care consultations, it is a nuisance. On an ongoing basis, practitioners will find it helpful to actively look out for resistance and move toward reducing it. This is not just a matter of what you say, or what strategy you use, but how you say it, and being in a flexible state of mind in which you *roll with resistance* (Miller and Rollnick, 2002) and avoid argument.

THREE TRAPS TO AVOID

Three traps have been isolated for particular attention, each giving rise to a strategy for avoiding it, described below. Fall into any of these traps and resistance will be a likely outcome.

TAKE CONTROL AWAY

We all know some patients who are very compliant and like to be told what to do. Most, however, do not respond well to this. Strategy 1 below (*emphasize personal choice and control*) illustrates how one can avoid this pitfall in a consultation.

MISJUDGE IMPORTANCE, CONFIDENCE, OR READINESS

This is a very common trap to fall into. For example, one can focus prematurely on change when the patient is not ready for this, or one could focus on importance when the patient is actually more concerned about confidence matters. Strategy 2 below (*reassess readiness, importance, and confidence*) involves reexamining the patient's feelings about these issues, to make sure that one remains aligned to his or her needs.

BOX 7.1 USEFUL QUESTIONS

Asking the patient questions is not the best way to reduce resistance. However, it will be *useful to ask yourself* these questions instead! Remember, resistance is an observable behavior (e.g., denial, reluctance). It can be influenced by the goals you pursue and by the way in which you speak to the patient.

1. Have you undermined the patient's sense of personal freedom? Can you hand this control back?
2. Have you misjudged the patient's feelings about readiness, importance, or confidence? Have you jumped too far ahead of the patient on these dimensions? Are you focusing on the wrong dimension? Consider how this patient really does feel about change.
3. Are you meeting force with force? Are you being too confrontational? Can you do anything to go along with the patient or even change tack altogether?

MEETING FORCE WITH FORCE

Whatever the topic of conversation and whoever the patient is, confronting resistance with force will make matters worse. A good consultation is not like a wrestling contest! However, use of Strategy 3 below (*back off and come alongside the patient*) will demonstrate that the rewards of avoiding confrontation are liberating, even though this is the most skillful of the strategies to execute.

WHAT TO AVOID

If the consultation begins to feel like a battle, and you feel as if you are going all out to win, there is a problem. People will defend themselves better the more they feel attacked. They will become deeper entrenched in their position. If you *do* win, will the patient feel they have lost? Is this the outcome you really want?

THREE STRATEGIES FOR REDUCING RESISTANCE

Three options described below are as follows:

- Emphasize personal choice and control
- Reassess readiness, importance, or confidence
- Back off and come alongside the patient

STRATEGY 1. EMPHASIZE PERSONAL CHOICE AND CONTROL

If a person is struggling to maintain some sense of control over his or her life, it does not take much to threaten this sense of stability. All one needs is a confrontation with a practitioner and resistance to change will emerge. It does not take much to fall into the trap of undermining the personal autonomy of the patient. Statements like *You should do…* or *The biggest problem you have is…* are likely to have this effect because they restrict the person's sense of freedom and will elicit resistance in the form of reassertion of autonomy (see Miron and Brehm, 2006). Every parent knows this problem; if you say to a young child, *You are dirty and you should go and wash now*, the almost instinctive reaction will be a form of resistance, which has more to do with personal autonomy being undermined than with the content of your statement. The content, for example, a response from the child like, *But I'm not dirty*, merely provides the stage on which the battle for autonomy is played out.

Practitioners, even when giving advice, appear to be well aware of these subtleties and apparently adjust their message accordingly, hence the discovery by Silverman (1997) that they make their advice ambiguous to avoid becoming too personal; they present their advice in neutral terms as if it is information. Another viable option to avoid threatening autonomy is to make this explicit. A simple phrase added on to a piece of advice can make all the difference: *I think that you should stop smoking now, but it's really up to you*. This might well avoid eliciting resistance. Leave out the second half and you could be in trouble.

It is also not merely a matter of *what* is being said but *how* it is being said. The practitioner's attitude and the atmosphere of the consultation will contribute to the patient's reaction. The same words used in two different atmospheres will have quite different effects.

A useful way of capturing the subtleties of this trap is to keep remembering that a confrontational interviewing style is likely to undermine autonomy and elicit resistance. This observation, which provided the starting point for motivational interviewing (see Miller, 1983), has been borne out in a number of studies which demonstrate that what happens in the consulting room affects patient outcome (Chamberlain et al., 1984; Miller and Sovereign, 1989). One study, for example, among help-seeking problem drinkers found that the number of confrontational statements made by counselors correlated with the amounts that patients drank at follow-up (Miller et al., 1993). The need to avoid confrontational interviewing provides the rationale for basing this approach on essential listening skills, which are the antithesis of confrontational interviewing. The spirit is more important than any strategy being employed (see chapter 2). The examples below illustrate this process of handing control back to the patient.

Many situations serve to undermine this sense of autonomy and are often associated with resistance to change. Handing this back to the patient can be done in many ways. Indeed, the assessment of readiness, importance, and confidence (Strategy 2) is one way of encouraging patients to return to saying exactly how they feel about change. Going through an agenda-setting exercise (Chapter 3) also has this goal as its explicit purpose.

If the patient is to be an active decision-maker, he or she must feel in control of choices that are made. These choices are about both what is talked about in the consultation and what the patient should do outside the consulting room.

Example 1

The patient attends a diabetes clinic for a routine check-up:

Practitioner: (After going through medical matters and feeding back the result of a blood test) And how's your food intake going?
Patient: OK.
Practitioner: How do you feel it is going? (Practitioner tries again)
Patient: Well, I try, but sometimes I break the rules, as you know.
Practitioner: I guessed that.
Patient: You see, it's been so busy, it's hard to always think about all this.
Practitioner: I can imagine. (Practitioner decides to shift focus and start again with agenda setting) Can we stand back from this for a moment and understand how you feel about the meeting today? What would you like to talk about today? We could talk about eating, exercise, your medication, or any of the usual things. But how do you feel? Perhaps there's something more pressing for you today that we could talk about? (See Chapter 3 for an outline of this strategy)
Patient: Well, one thing I do know is that…

Example 2

The patient says they've come for a *diet sheet*:

Practitioner: You say you would like some dietary advice. Have I ever shown you this record sheet? The idea is that you keep a record on a daily basis for the next week.
Patient: No, but I've tried that sort of thing once before. It was just hopeless. (Resistance)
Practitioner: I understand. I wonder what you think will be most helpful to you?
Patient: Well, what I need to do is to be able to…

Example 3

In this next example, the patient's sense of control over a heart attack is delicately balanced and unwittingly undermined by the practitioner's action talk. Once again, the practitioner tries to give control over what is talked about in the consultation to the patient.

Practitioner: (Aiming to build confidence about behavior change) So these exercises are specially designed to help someone like you who has had a heart attack, to help you slowly get back on your feet again.
Patient: OK, thanks. (Little conviction)
Practitioner: You can do them once a day to start off with, perhaps soon after you get up in the morning.
Patient: Uhmmm. (Possible resistance)
Practitioner: (Wondering whether the above apparent agreement is, in fact, resistance) There's something worrying you about doing that.

Patient: Well, how do I know that I won't have another heart attack?
Practitioner: You think, perhaps, that too much exercise might make things worse.
Patient: Well, that's right, couldn't it?
Practitioner: (Realizes that there is something else of greater concern to the patient) Do you think we should chat for a minute or two about the risk and that sort of thing? (Shifting focus to information exchange)
Patient: Well, you can't help wondering when it's going to happen again.
Practitioner: How do you understand what is happening to your heart? (First phase of information exchange, i.e., elicit the patient's understanding)

In this example, the practitioner made a decision to focus on confidence-building, but the patient was more concerned about something else. The control over what was to be discussed was not given to the patient to begin with. The observation of resistance provided the basis for the practitioner's decision-making in the consultation, to shift focus from a confidence-building strategy to an information exchange strategy, one that in this case assumed less readiness to change. By understanding the source of this resistance, *There's something worrying you about doing that*, the practitioner was able to find a task (information exchange) that was congruent with the needs of the patient and gave him or her greater control over what was talked about and any decision-making about behavior change.

STRATEGY 2. REASSESS READINESS, IMPORTANCE, OR CONFIDENCE

A common cause of resistance is when the practitioner falls into the trap of overestimating or misjudging readiness, importance, or confidence. Most often, this results in premature action talk. If readiness is seen as a continuum and the patient is at the not-ready end, practitioner talk which assumes that the patient either is or should be at the ready end (action talk) will elicit resistance. Seen in this light, resistance is a measure of the extent to which the practitioner has jumped ahead of the patient. The obvious practical implication is that a shift in the practitioner's strategy is necessary to reestablish congruence with the patient's state of readiness. The same overestimation mistake can be made when the talk is about either the importance of change or the confidence to achieve it. For example, a practitioner establishes that a smoker would very much like to give up (i.e., importance is high), but the smoker is concerned about achieving this (i.e., confidence is low). The practitioner makes the mistake of assuming that confidence should be higher and more amenable to shifting than it really is and that a few bits of simple advice on how to go about it will suffice. Some suggestions are offered. The outcome is resistance.

This discussion has assumed that the patient would like to talk about behavior change. However, a more dramatic, yet very common, example of overestimation is to focus on behavior change when the patient is more concerned about something else. Thus the exercise specialist talks about exercise when a patient in cardiac rehabilitation is feeling depressed and fearful about having another episode of myocardial ischemia, or the patient attending a diabetes clinic is in a hurry to get shopping and does not wish to talk about diet.

A practitioner can also misjudge (rather than overestimate) a patient's feelings by focusing on confidence instead of importance or vice versa. This is a common mistake to make. Might this be the problem with the husband described at the beginning of this chapter, who is actually not convinced about the importance of change, while the discussion focuses on confidence? People often come into action-orientated clinics and slip into talk about practical measures to improve confidence to change. Health-care practitioners are trained to do things to people and to solve problems. When they attend seminars on particular health behavior topics, they are hungry for more ideas on what to suggest to their patients to help them to change.

If you have made the mistake of either overestimating one of these qualities or focusing on the wrong one, the most obvious response to the resistance that can arise is to reevaluate the direction you are taking. This can be done explicitly by asking the patient to tell you how he or she really feels, particularly about the distinction between importance and confidence. This can be achieved in a few minutes.

This reassessment does not necessarily have to be done in an explicit manner but can be achieved simply by sharing with the patient your confusion about what exactly his or her concerns are. Here is an example of what one might say to someone reluctant to become more active.

Practitioner: How do you feel about being more active?
Patient: I'd like to, yes.
Practitioner: Have you thought about what kind of activity suits you?
Patient: It's not so easy for me. I hate sports and competition; I never did like that sort of thing.
Practitioner: What about walking? (Practitioner tries to focus on confidence-building)
Patient: It's not safe where I live. I come off my shift late at night and it's madness out there… These kids are wild, like they just don't care about anyone.
Practitioner: And a gym? (Is the practitioner still focusing on confidence instead of importance?)
Patient: I can't afford that sort of thing.
Practitioner: (Does he feel that exercise is not really that important to him? A decision is made to see whether the talk about confidence is a mistake. This could be done explicitly by asking the patient to rate importance and confidence on a scale of 1–10, but on this occasion, the shifting of gear in the face of resistance is done more subtly) I'm not sure what to think. Perhaps you are feeling that there's no easy solution here and that there are other things that are more important to you right now than getting more exercise.
Patient: Well, you know what I mean, sometimes one just has to put up with what life throws at you, like I've got a lot going on at the moment and who knows how I can get more exercise.

Practitioner: It's hard to see how to fit it all in.
Patient: That's right, I'm not a perfect machine; I'm more like a reliable old car…
Practitioner: Maybe now's not the time for a tune-up.
Patient: Who knows, I don't really know what to do.
Practitioner: So, in some ways you'd like to be more active, and at the same time, there are lots of obstacles to fitting it into your life and you're not sure if it's worth it.
Patient: Well, I know both the wife and myself have become quite lazy over the years, and it would do us both good if…

STRATEGY 3. BACK OFF AND COME ALONGSIDE THE PATIENT

This strategy is designed to counter the trap of meeting force with force. It captures this heart of motivational interviewing, i.e., responding to resistance by keeping in a state of mind in which one does not "take the bait" or meet force with force but goes along with the patient. The technique of making reflective listening statements is a direct way of achieving this.

The spirit in which this strategy is conducted is important. Avoiding argument is not just a passive process in which one sits back in a defensive posture and uses reflective listening until the fire dies down but one in which the practitioner tries to come alongside the patient and truly understand how he or she is feeling. If successful, the resistance will usually subside, and the discussion can move in a different direction.

The technique of reflective listening has its roots in the client-centered therapy of Carl Rogers (1951). It involves making statements designed to show that you understand the meaning of what the person is saying (see Miller and Rollnick, 2002). The effect of using such statements, as opposed to questions, is to encourage the patient to continue talking and expressing his or her views and feelings. Fig. 2.4 on p. 38 can be a useful aid for understanding this process. The reflective statements can take a variety of forms: repeating exactly what the person has said, rephrasing it in different words, or adding new meaning to that expressed by the patient. These statements often begin with words like *so you…, you feel…, it's as if…* and *you…*

In this example, the entire sequence is characterized by the use of reflective listening. We are not implying that questions are not useful but simply want to illustrate how far one can go with reflective listening. In reality, one might use a fair proportion of questions and summary statements. The goal of coming alongside the patient is what matters.

Practitioner: I wonder what would suit you best, to look at your eating or to think about taking more exercise? (Opening question)
Patient: I get as much exercise as I want, and every time I try to diet, I end up eating the fried foods that the kids get. (Resistance)

Practitioner: You don't want to try something that's not going to work. (A reflective listening statement that aligns practitioner with patient and does not increase the resistance)

Patient: That's right, if I could do something with the diet, I would.

Practitioner: You can't see a way forward on this one at the moment. (Another reflection)

Patient: But what if I carry on the way I am?

A CASE EXAMPLE OF REDUCING RESISTANCE

Occasionally, people come into the consulting room feeling very defensive and irritable. The potential for a serious inflammation is obvious. This next example illustrates how going along with the person and using reflective listening can build rapport and avoid serious conflict. It is a verbatim transcript of a simulated encounter between Pip Mason playing a practitioner and a professional actor in the role of a pregnant mother (Gilligan and Mason, 2008). Neither party was prepared beforehand about how the consultation would proceed. The practitioner has conducted the routine "preliminary" interview and raises the subject of smoking.

Practitioner: We're offering a service now to any of our pregnant moms who want to give up smoking. Am I right in thinking you're smoking at the moment? (Raises the issue)

Sarah: (Crosses arms) Well, yes.

Practitioner: Can you tell me a bit about that and how you feel about it? (Open question)

Sarah: I wondered when we were going to get on to this to be honest. Well, I am a smoker and I smoked through my last three pregnancies. My babies were absolutely fine and as I've told you, they're all happy, healthy children. So in that sense, I don't think there's anything for me to worry about.

Practitioner: So it seems to you that although other people go on about it, they are probably making a bit of a fuss about it. (Reflection of the resistance)

Sarah: Yes, I think people see me and they just want to find something to criticize and, to be honest, my family are really happy and healthy and I am and—you've seen from my health check I'm in good health and Joe is too—I just think it's one of those things that should be a matter of personal choice.

Practitioner: So you must be wondering why we keep asking about it and want to keep talking about it. (More reflection of resistance)

Sarah: Well, I know, of course, you read things in magazines and so on, there are some dangers and I understand that, and that's why you've got to do your job, but I think when you weigh up all the pros and the cons, I don't think it's that big a deal.

Practitioner: (Nods) So when you talk about personal choice, it would be quite important to you to carry on smoking, it's something you value. (Reflects resistance and opens up topic of importance)

Sarah: Well, I wouldn't say it's something I value, because… it's not like I'm proud that I'm a smoker… it just helps me… having three kids, it can be really stressful and sometimes I think if I didn't have just those few minutes a day to have a cigarette and a bit of time to myself, I don't think I'd be as good a mother as I am.

Practitioner: Uh huh… you think you'd get more stressed out. (Reflection of the cons of change)

Sarah: Definitely, I know I would and I've seen other people do it… I've seen some friends of mine… and my Mom… when she tried to stop, she was a nightmare. I'm not exaggerating and I don't want to put my family through that.

Practitioner: So you think one of the hardest things if you were to give up would be getting stressed. If you didn't have that outlet for yourself. (Reflection of resistance)

Sarah: Yeah, definitely, I just can't see how I could do that.

Practitioner: What other things would be difficult for you?

Sarah: Well, it would be really hard because Joe smokes. That would be really hard if I managed to stop and he didn't. We'd be sitting there when the kids have gone to bed watching the TV and he's having a smoke. I just can't see how that would work.

Practitioner: Yes, I can see that would be hard. (Empathic statement)

Sarah: Yes, it would be.

Practitioner: And what other things?

Sarah: I mean, on the one hand, I know that it's obvious in a way but things are quite tight money-wise at the moment with a fourth baby on the way that wasn't exactly planned, and if we both stopped, that would be one thing, we'd have a bit more money, but I worry we'd be so unhappy that it wouldn't do us any favors.

Practitioner: So although it's costing you a lot of money, you think it might be worth it. What is it that makes it worth spending that money, for you? (Inquires about pros of smoking)

Sarah: It's part of me, I am a smoker, me and Joe, we met when we were kids and he was smoking when I met him and then I started just after that when I was about 15 and that's just who we are.

Practitioner: Yeah, part of your own identity and your identity as a couple. (Reflection)

Sarah: Yeah, I can't imagine, it's part of unwinding, having a drink and a cigarette.

Practitioner: But it sounds as if you've thought about it a bit. You've thought about how difficult it would be, which suggests from time to time you've wondered about doing it. (Reflection)

Sarah: Yeah, I mean it's always come up when I've seen midwives about having the kids. I was anxious about it with you coming today, getting nagged about it. But I've thought about it and I did try once, in my second pregnancy… and I made it for a day but then the next day went back and for me, I thought what's the point? If I couldn't do it then, I'm not going to be able to now.

Practitioner: You don't think you've any chance. (Reflection)

Sarah: Not really.

Practitioner: So if I asked you on a scale of 1—10 if you wanted to give up (and I hear what you're saying that you don't know if you want to…), if you did want to, how confident are you that you could? It sounds as if it might be quite low. (Begins to explore confidence)

Sarah: To be honest, I'd probably say about a 2.

Practitioner: But not a 1! I thought you were going to give me a 1 or 0. Is there a little bit of you, perhaps, that thinks you might be able to do it? (Variation on *Why so high?* question)

Sarah: Well. I am a strong person you see…

In this interview, the practitioner raises the issue, detects resistance, and uses a reflective style to roll with resistance. Confidence emerges as an issue, and the health practitioner uses a scaling question to encourage Sarah to talk positively about herself as someone who might be able to change.

CONCLUSION

We have covered three traps in this discussion of resistance. There are undoubtedly others that the practitioner can fall into which lead to resistance. These are merely the most commonly occurring ones that we have come across. For example, what if the patient wants more or less direction than the practitioner is offering? This is one of the most puzzling and challenging aspects of behavior change consultations, which is discussed in more detail in Chapter 11. A mismatch of this kind is likely to lead to resistance. Clearly, more work needs to be done on this issue.

Awareness of strategies for dealing with resistance should not overshadow the most important guideline: *watch, look, and listen*. If you meet resistance, change tack. Simply being aware of it, and not making it worse, often leads quite directly into the use of strategies outlined below, sometimes quite unconsciously. This is certainly not just a technical matter of using this or that strategy but of being in a watchful and flexible frame of mind and remembering that you do not have to feel responsible for providing a counterargument. Resistance is often a signal for you to change gear and to repair damaged rapport, usually by going along with patients and talking in a way more in sympathy with their feelings and attitudes. Be watchful for the patient who is in verbal accord with you but whose body language demonstrates the opposite.

The challenge for practitioners is first to develop awareness of resistance and then to practice being flexible in response to it to maintain a lightness of touch that allows them to avoid meeting force with counterargument. Resistance is a key to successful treatment if you can recognize it for the opportunity that it is. In expressing resistance, the patient is probably rehearsing a script that has been played out many times before. There is an expected role for you to play — one that has been acted out by others in the past. Your lines are predictable. If you speak these same lines, as others have done, the script will come to the same conclusion as before. But you can rewrite your own role. You can witness the patient's internal conflict rather than joining in to advocate change.

Resistance lies at the heart of the interplay. It arises from the motives and struggles of the actors. It foreshadows certain ends to which the play may or may not lead. The true art of therapy is tested in the recognition and handling of resistance. It is on this stage that the drama of change unfolds (Miller and Rollnick 2002, p. 110).

KEY POINTS

- Resistance is a normal response from someone who feels they are being put under pressure.
- Empathy is a better way to reduce resistance than confrontation.
- Argument and confrontation tend to increase resistance.

REFERENCES

Bradley, C.P., 1992. Uncomfortable prescribing decisions: a critical incident study. British Medical Journal 304, 294–296.

Brehm, J.W., 1966. A Theory of Psychological Reactance. Academic Press, New York, NY.

Butler, C.C., Rollnick, S., Pill, R., Maggs-Rapport, F., Stott, N., 1998. Understanding the culture of prescribing: a qualitative study of general practitioners' and patients' perceptions of antibiotics for sore throats. British Medical Journal 317, 637–642.

Chamberlain, O., Patterson, G., Reid, J., Kavanagh, K., Forgatch, M., 1984. Observation of client resistance. Behavior Therapy 15, 144–155.

Egan, G., 1994. The Skilled Helper: A Problem Management Approach to Helping. Brooks/Cole, Pacific Grove.

Gilligan, T., Mason, P., 2008. Engaging Motivation 2 (DVD). Pip Mason Consultancy Ltd, Birmingham.

Miller, W.R., 1983. Motivational interviewing with problem drinkers. Behavioral Psychotherapy 1, 147–172.

Miller, W.R., Sovereign, R., 1989. The check-up: a model for early intervention in addictive behaviors. In: Loberg, T., Miller, W.R., Nathan, P.E., Marlatt, G.A. (Eds.), Addictive Behaviors: Prevention and Early Intervention. Swets & Zeitlinger, Amsterdam.

Miller, W., Benefield, R., Tonigan, S., 1993. Enhancing motivation for change in problem drinking: a controlled comparison of two therapist styles. Journal of Consulting and Clinical Psychology 61, 455–461.

Miller, W.R., Rollnick, S., 2002. Motivational Interviewing: Preparing People for Change, second ed. Guilford Press, New York.

Miller, W.R., Rollnick, S., 2012. Motivational Interviewing: Helping People Change, third ed. Guilford Press, New York.

Miron, A.M., Brehm, J.W., 2006. Reactance theory — 40 years later. Zeitschrift Für Sozialpsychologie 9—18. https://doi.org/10.1024/0044-3514.37.1.9.

Rogers, C.R., 1951. Client-Centred Therapy. Houghton Mifflin, Boston.

Silverman, D., 1997. Discourses in Counselling: HIV Counselling as Social Interaction. Sage, London.

Ending the consultation

INTRODUCTION

> I haven't really looked at it like that before. I need to go away and think about it some more before I make a decision about what to do.
>
> I understand what you're saying and I know you're probably right but I just can't see my way to doing it at the moment.

Consultations do not always have happy endings, with the patient going away with a clear action plan. When we are aware that our time for this meeting is running out, it can be tempting to try and push toward action to finish things up neatly. However, to do so is to run the risk of raising resistance, as the patient feels pressurized. Have you ever been considering buying a jacket and ended up leaving the shop without it because an over-pushy sales assistant tried to make the sale while you were still thinking about it? Or, have you ever considered a major purchase and

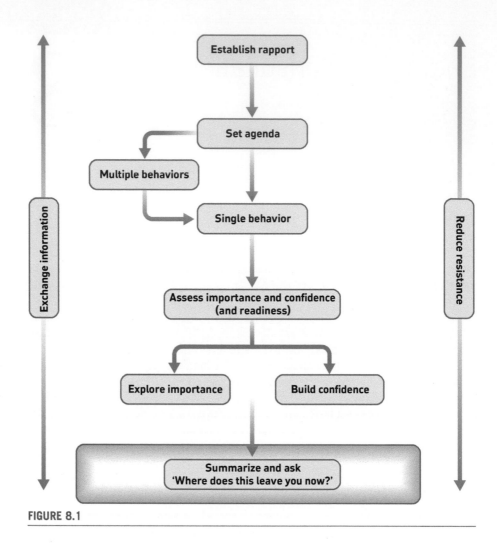

FIGURE 8.1

then gone home to sleep on the decision before committing yourself? Hasty decisions are not always the best ones.

Our consultations are short. However, the journey toward change may be long. Early in the previous century, children would play a game bowling hoops along the road. The hoop had an impetus of its own. Its natural inclination was to roll along. Occasionally, it needed a nudge from the child to keep it on track or stop it falling over. Our consultations might be like the child's nudge: helpful from time to time, but the real momentum for change is in the patient. Consequently, each consultation might be seen as one fragment of an overall process, rather than a discrete event. So what we need is a way of closing the session without closing the process. We may need to free ourselves from the assumption that a good consultation has to finish with a positive action plan. We do not have to "close the sale" as they say in marketing.

A good way to move toward closing the consultation is to summarize the discussion so far and to ask an open question along the lines of, *Where does this leave you now?* The patient's answer will tell you where to go next.

I can see it's important but there are other things I think I need to prioritize at the moment. [Not ready to change]

I need to give this some more thought and talk it through with my family. [Still unsure]

I can see it makes sense for me to do it. What's the best way to go about it? Where do we go from here? [Ready to change]

WHAT TO AVOID

The practitioner wants to be able to continue dialogue on this issue in future sessions. Three bad outcomes are as follows: first, if the patient goes away with a hastily constructed and unrealistic action plan, fails to keep to it and is embarrassed to come back and admit it. Second, it is unhelpful if the patient goes away feeling nagged and judged, and next time they need help, they feel reluctant to come and see us (or even decide to change practitioner) because we keep trying to get them to change. Third, we will not do our best by them if we diagnose reluctant patients as being "in pre-contemplation" and write them off, not bothering to raise the topic with them again.

PATIENT NOT READY TO CHANGE

It is difficult to feel positive when someone has not made their mind up to change by the time the consultation ends. It is even more difficult, perhaps, when they have made a clear decision not to change! Practitioners know they have to respect their decision, but what does that really mean?

It does not mean we have to like it. On occasions, we may feel genuinely sad that they do not feel ready to do something that we think would be really helpful to them. We may feel exasperated because their continuing poor health or risk-taking will make more work for their families and for us. It means accepting that it really is their life and they absolutely have the right to make their own decisions about which risks to take and how to live. People risks their health through obesity because they love fatty food; another risks injury by spending their holidays downhill skiing because the danger itself makes it exhilarating. The practitioner's role is to ensure, as far as we are able, that these decisions are informed and thoughtful.

In some circumstances, we have a harm-reduction role with patients who do not make healthy choices. We may treat smokers' lung infections and discuss with them keeping their home smoke-free for the children, and we may medicate high blood pressure in patients who do not wish to make the lifestyle changes that would bring it down.

> **BOX 8.1 USEFUL QUESTIONS**
> 1. Where does this leave you now?
> 2. What would it be helpful for you to do between now and when we meet again?
> 3. What's your next step?
> 4. Is there any information you'd like me to give you that would help you make your mind up about this?
> 5. What have you learned from previous attempts to change? What does your experience tell you about the best way to go about this?

It can be interesting to ask, *What would need to happen for you to reconsider change?* Such a question can keep the topic on the agenda. Reflecting the answer can help the patient to pay attention to what they are saying and to check they are comfortable with the decision.

Practitioner: So, on the one hand you feel you ought to stop smoking because of your health and to protect your children. However, you are not ready to do so yet. So you are going to continue smoking for the time being. What would it take for you to reconsider this decision? Is there anything that might happen in the next year or two that would change your mind?

Patient: Well… I suppose if one of my kids actually got ill as a direct result of my smoking…

Practitioner: [Reflects] So you're not ready to quit yet and you'll probably carry on until, eventually, if your smoking actually makes one of the children ill, that might make you think about it again.

Patient: I suppose that is what I'm saying, hmmm…

If patients feel that their decisions and their right to make them are respected, it is more likely that they will feel comfortable coming back for help if they do reconsider in the future. You have given them a taste of what to expect; they know they will not be judged or bullied and that they will be helped to find their own way through. The door is left open.

PATIENT STILL UNSURE

Sometimes, the patient has not so much decided against change as been given a lot to think about which will take time to process. In some ways, it is important to them to change but is it important enough to sacrifice what they will lose? They have some belief in their ability to do it but this falls short of confidence. They need to go away and think some more, and this is what we should help them to do.

The decisional balance sheet (Table 5.2 on p. 84) can help patients to focus. You may have used it with them already, but taking it home to think about may generate more clarity. Family members might add to it too if the topic is appropriate for sharing. If you have an ongoing relationship with the patient, you can ask when you see them again: *Did you have any more thoughts about X after we talked last time?* Being given well-chosen information to take away may also help, remembering the *elicit—provide—elicit* strategy from Chapter 6.

PATIENT READY TO CHANGE

Many consultations will reach the point where the patient decides to make the change. Once the decision is made, the next step is action planning. This might be simple: for example, changing a medication. It might be complicated: for example, designing a diet for weight loss. It might need to be put off until a further appointment or a referral may need to be made to someone else with expertise in the area. The principle of empowering the patient remains.

- As far as possible, allow the patient to generate ideas. If they need help, offer them a menu of ideas you know have worked for other people, and encourage them to choose the one that will work for them.
- Exchange information on the process of making this particular change (e.g., information on common experiences of cravings and withdrawals when giving up smoking, reasonable expectations of weight loss when committing to a healthy eating program).
- Watch for resistance. In your enthusiasm to move toward action, you may be tempted to move too fast. Patients' reactions will give you feedback on this. If you are jumping ahead of them, slow down: *Maybe now you've made the decision, you'd rather give yourself a bit of time to think about how you can best go about it.*

Ask, before they go, *What's your next step?* In motivational interviewing, it is seen as important to elicit *change talk* from the patient. The strongest form of change talk is *commitment*. If the patient hears him- or herself say something like *The first thing I'm going to do when I get home is…* or *I need to get the ball rolling so the first step is to…* and if they commit to taking a step in the right direction soon after leaving you, they will be more likely to make the plan happen.

HOW DO I KNOW IF I HAVE DONE A GOOD JOB?

Sometimes you will do a brilliant job, following all the guidelines for good practice and for forging an excellent helping alliance with the patient, and the outcome is that the patient decides change is not for him or her. Other times, you will clumsily muddle your way through a consultation and the patient will go away enthusiastically with an action plan to which they feel committed! The first might have been a proficient piece of work with a disappointing outcome, and the second, a poor piece of practice with the best possible result. Although we are interested in "success rates" in population terms, in our clinical experience, we cannot totally equate our own performance with the decisions that our patients make.

However, as reflective practitioners, we all want to take stock every now and again and appraise our work, so it may be helpful to have some questions to ask ourselves.

WHO DID MOST OF THE TALKING IN THAT ENCOUNTER?

When using this approach, the patient does most of the talking. Even when the practitioner is talking, much of what they are saying is reflection and summarizing what the patient said. When you look back on a consultation, does it feel as if you gave them a "good talking to" or was it rather a "good listening to"?

CAN YOU NOW SUMMARIZE THEIR MAIN CONCERNS AND ASPIRATIONS IN RELATION TO CHANGE?

Here's a test of whether you were really listening. Can you describe their world? Have you understood what they were trying to tell you? Have you heard what is important to them, or were you focusing more on your own priorities?

DID YOU GIVE THEM THE OPPORTUNITY TO RECEIVE ANY INFORMATION THAT MIGHT HAVE AFFECTED THEIR DECISION?

Whatever decision they made, was it an informed one? Or, at least, did you offer the information? Although in this approach, the listening is emphasized more than the talking, our duty of care to patients means that we have a responsibility to check and update their information base when helping them to make decisions.

WAS IT CLEAR TO BOTH OF YOU THAT RESPONSIBILITY FOR CHANGE LIES WITH THE PATIENT?

When you reflect back on the consultation, what messages did your language convey about responsibility? Did you say *Our options are…* or was it *Your options are…*? If the patient showed reluctance or resistance, did you emphasize their personal control: *Well it is your decision, it's your call on this one…*, or did you try and talk them into your option? Most importantly, perhaps, were you then, and are you now, clear in your own mind about where your responsibilities begin and end?

WHAT IF THE CHANGE DOES NOT LAST?

If you work hard, the patient makes a determined, robust decision to change, does really well for a while and then slips back into old habits; this tells you something really important about them. They are normal! The journey to long-lasting lifestyle change typically passes through a series of temporary attempts, some more successful than others. Each is an opportunity to learn more about what helps or hinders the journey for this particular patient. Prochaska et al. (1994) report that only 5% of people they followed for 2 years made it through the change process without at least one setback. They refer to the *spiral of change* and talk about *recycling* rather than *relapse*. Instead of "going back to square one," people quickly move into preparing for the next attempt, incorporating lessons learned from recent experiences and mistakes.

However, it is all very well to be philosophical about it in principle. In practice, it can really feel like failure, even if we are careful to avoid the word. It is disappointing to put weight back on that was lost or to be smoking again after experiencing a smoke-free life for a while. Family members may feel let down. If the consultations were part of a program for which we have been set outcome targets, we may be disappointed and frustrated. It may be most helpful to acknowledge these feelings before moving on to a more positive approach to picking up the pieces and starting again. An analogy might be the child who is learning to ride a bike and falls off. She needs a little cry and a cuddle before getting back on bravely for another go.

Practitioner: You sound quite disappointed that you've put on so much of the weight that you lost earlier in the year.

Patient: Yes, I really thought I'd cracked it this time, and I looked and felt so much better.

Practitioner: It gave you a taste of how things could be different.

Patient: It did. It feels really hard to have to start again, but I suppose if I've done it once, I can do it again.

Practitioner: Well, if it is still important to you and you decide to give it another try, there might be lots we can both learn about what worked well and what worked less well last time.

Some relapses are very clear-cut, such as the smoker who ends a period of abstinence by deciding to smoke again and buying a pack of cigarettes and a lighter. The decision to smoke again was deliberate and a conscious action. Other relapses are more insidious, such as the person who drops his or her gym visits from four times a week to just the weekends because of work and then seems to miss lots of weekend sessions because of other commitments and eventually becomes quite inactive while still having an image of themselves as someone who goes to the gym. It can be helpful to follow up change in one way or another to nudge things back on course and draw the patient's attention to any unintentional slippage.

It can be important not to push people prematurely into another attempt. In smoking cessation services, it is common to suggest that people who have relapsed should wait a few weeks or months before another quit attempt. Trying again before they are really ready can lead to more relapse, and although it can be turned into a learning experience, too many relapses can be overwhelming and demoralizing. The key task in helping someone get back on course after a relapse is usually confidence-building. However, some relapses occur because, owing to other events in the person's life, the behavior change has become less important and they need to reevaluate whether it is a priority just now.

KEY POINTS

- The situation might not be resolved in one session and that is OK. If the patient leaves with something to think about and that can be a good, realistic outcome for a single brief intervention.
- When moving into action, it is important to maintain the spirit of patient choice and empowerment. Prescription risks resistance.
- Change is usually a journey, not an event.
- Relapse is normal and not usually the end of the journey.

REFERENCE

Prochaska, J.O., Norcross, J.C., Diclemente, C.C., 1994. Changing for Good. William Morrow, New York.

Common clinical encounters

CHAPTER OUTLINE

Previous chapters have described our approach to various tasks in a consultation that could involve attention to patient behavior. The aim of this chapter is to illustrate this approach by taking examples from a range of clinical settings. Because of the striking uniformity in talk about behavior change, these strategies should be widely applicable. The same topics of conversation arise again and again. However, there is also remarkable diversity, where each encounter is a unique conversation in which a practitioner must adapt the strategy to suit the situation. The clinical scenarios below are not intended to be models of good practice but illustrations of how a practitioner can use the toolbox in a range of situations.

TALKING ABOUT SMOKING
TYPICAL SCENARIOS

You are a primary care practitioner. A patient has bronchitis and requests antibiotics. You know she is a heavy smoker.

You are a nurse conducting a chronic disease management clinic. A person with hypertension or diabetes attends for review; his condition is not well controlled, and he continues to smoke.

GOALS

- To make the most of the "teachable moment" when the presenting health problem or an established health problem is directly connected to unhealthy behaviors.
- To provide the structure for patients to identify goals for themselves.
- To ensure that goals are realistic and build on the patient's resources for change.
- To maximize intrinsic motivation and to harness the patient's own ideas and resources for change.
- To realize that smoking is a major addiction that is influenced by a complex web of personal and social factors and which is only very rarely overcome as a result of one brief consultation. Goals for the behavior change aspect of this

consultation will vary according to the importance that individual patients place on change and their confidence in their ability to see it through. Simply planting a seed for change is a worthy achievement.

- To avoid alienating patients by giving them yet another unwelcome lecture that repeats what they have heard many times before.
- To avoid setting impossible goals so that the patient will inevitably harbor a sense of failure and frustration when he or she next consults.
- To avoid being left frustrated by attempting to "police" patients and failing to "get people to change."
- To provide the structure for individual patients to make effective decisions rather than trying to live their lives for them.

PRINCIPLES AND STRATEGIES

- Raise the subject in a nonthreatening way by affirming your goal of understanding patients' perspectives and respect for their decisions, even if these run counter to best medical wisdom.
- Explore how important giving up smoking is to patients, and build their confidence in their ability to succeed in giving up.
- If importance is low, focus on that through asking useful scaling questions about the importance score.
- Explore importance further by asking about pros and cons of smoking.
- Offer to share information in a nonjudgmental way with those for whom giving up is not important. Keep the door open.
- Where giving up is important to patients but their confidence in succeeding is low, hone in on perceived barriers. Try the useful scaling questions about increasing confidence.
- Ask patients to take you through a typical day in their lives, as this will enhance rapport. Invite patients to make their own judgments about how they view the smoking.
- Brainstorm solutions to overcoming the barriers to successful quitting that are identified by patients themselves.
- Negotiate attainable goals.
- Agree to a follow-up.

POSSIBLE PRACTICE

Practitioner: Yes, I agree you have bronchitis again. But it would help me get a better picture of your chest and your health more generally if we could take a few minutes to talk about your smoking. I'm certainly not going to give you yet another lecture. I know you have had more than one or two of those! Today, my goal is to really try to understand a bit more about smoking from your viewpoint. OK? Won't you tell me what sort of smoker you are?

[The patient responds, usually briefly]

Practitioner: I'm going to ask you two questions now that will help me understand things more clearly, and I want you to rate your answers on a scale. First, how important is giving up smoking to you right now? If 1 is "not at all important" and 10 is "very important," what number would you give yourself right now?
[The patient thinks for a moment and gives a number]

Practitioner: OK, great. Now I want to ask you about your confidence in your ability to quit and remain a nonsmoker. If you did decide to try and quit, and 1 is "not at all confident" and 10 is "very confident" that you could give up and stay a nonsmoker, what number would you give yourself now?

If importance is low, ask a question like *You gave yourself a 3 for importance to you of giving up smoking. Why not 1?* Whatever basis there is for the patient's motivation to change will now emerge, such as *I can't afford to smoke so much, I know it's bad for me.* This has been called *change talk* (Miller and Rollnick, 2012).

If confidence is the main problem, either of these kinds of questions can be asked for confidence. An additional useful question is: *What can I, or we in this clinic, do to help you move up from a 3 to a 6 or 7?*

When low importance is the main problem, the patient is usually feeling ambivalent; asking about the pros and cons of smoking may bring aspects of the patient's dilemma into sharp focus. The heightened tension from making the ambivalence so explicit may prompt serious consideration about change.

Building on the notion that it is better for patients to make their own evaluations about how their behavior affects them and how they should respond, the practitioner invites the patient to say what he or she likes and dislikes about the behavior in question. After the patient has listed the positive sides, the practitioner, without interrupting or interpreting, asks the patient to list the negative side of the coin as he or she sees it. The practitioner attempts to summarize both the pros and cons of the dilemma, keeping as close as possible to the words used by the patient, and then asks the patient to say how the summary leaves him or her feeling and thinking. Practitioners should fight hard to avoid capitulating to inevitable urges to push their own health-care agenda.

Practitioner: Tell me what you like about smoking.

Patient: You really want to know what I like about smoking? Most people I've seen just give me the hell and damnation bit. Well now, let's see, smoking definitely helps me relax, and in my job with all the uncertainty, I need that. I live a very stressful life you know. Funnily enough, smoking also gives me a feeling of giving something to myself, like it's my time for me. And I enjoy having a smoke when I have a drink with my friends.

Practitioner: OK, now tell me what you dislike about smoking?

Patient: Well, my wife nags me to hell and back, that's for certain. It does stink a bit, my kids hate it, and sometimes I do worry about what it's doing to my lungs…

Practitioner: OK. So, on the one hand, you've got a stressful job and smoking gives you time for yourself, it helps you to relax and socialize. On the other hand, it stinks, your family gives you a hard time about it, and sometimes you get worried about what it's doing to your health. Have I got it more or less about right? OK. Now, where does that leave you feeling right now about your smoking?

Patient: Well, it certainly is a problem. I guess I've got to sit down and do some hard thinking.

Another useful strategy is the Typical Day strategy, where the practitioner asks the patient to think of a recent, typical day in his or her life and talk the practitioner through it, mentioning where the smoking fits in and how they felt about it. Again, the practitioner avoids the temptation to interrupt and extract lessons; the process of self-articulation is often a much more powerful teacher than external proselytizing. It also helps to build rapport and engenders an understanding of the patient as a person. This interpersonal understanding and consequent sense of mutual respect can be a very powerful therapeutic tool.

For those patients for whom giving up smoking is not important right now, avoid nihilism. Sometimes exploring ambivalence among patients who seem really set against change brings startling success. This is precisely the group that is least likely to receive opportunistic health promotion (Sesney et al., 1997).

Offer to share information in a nonjudgmental way:

Sure, it sounds like you are not ready to really stop right now. That's fine. It's your decision and after all, no one else can make decisions for you. But I was just wondering whether some up-to-date medical information about the effects of smoking and perhaps some of the new treatments might help you in your decision-making.

Endeavor to couch information in general terms and then ask the patient to provide interpretations about his or her own specific circumstances:

The research clearly shows that smoking does more damage among people with diabetes than those who do not have diabetes. On average, a 50-year-old smoker with diabetes will live an extra 3 years if he or she were to give up smoking. I wonder what you make of that?

Many patients will say that they already know all they want to know about the ill effects of smoking. As a rule, smokers are well informed about the negative health consequences of smoking, and a qualitative interview study we conducted shows that established smokers feel that they have already been saturated with antismoking information (Butler et al., 1998). The practitioner may respond to this:

Fine, OK, you know as much about the good and the bad sides of smoking as you feel you need to know. But can we agree to keep the door open on this one? Things often change and if you want to discuss the issue at any time, feel free to get in touch. By the way, did you hear about that woman in France who suddenly decided to give up smoking at the age of 112?

For patients who feel that it is important to give up but who are low in confidence to succeed, *brainstorming solutions* can identify practical ways forward which are meaningful to the patient's unique situation. Say a patient identifies fear of weight gain as the main barrier to giving up smoking. The practitioner may ask her to identify broad approaches to tackling this particular stumbling block. For example, one might ask, *What things do you know that people can do to lose weight?* Again, the practitioner encourages the patient to provide solutions and interpretations before offering suggestions of his or her own. Various general topic areas are identified: for example, exercise, diet, drugs, eating less, eating differently, weight loss programs, and so on. The practitioner then asks, *Does any of these approaches appeal to you at the present time?* Again, patients can be encouraged to choose the approach that suits them best. They might say, *Yes well, I could try eating differently.* The practitioner again avoids jumping in with suggestions like *Stop eating fast food meals* or *Don't fry your food* and instead asks the patient to identify possibilities. Creative and surprising suggestions frequently emerge that practitioners might never have thought of in a 1000 years but which patients come up with immediately.

Giving lectures that set impossible goals for patients condemns both practitioners and patients to inevitable failure: *I've told you before, and I am going to tell you again. By the time I next see you, you simply must have given up smoking, be eating only salads, have stopped drinking so much, and have started an exercise and relaxation program.* Not likely! It is incumbent on the practitioner to ensure that the goals that patients select to work on are short term and attainable; most patients with unhealthy behaviors have taken years to get into their present predicament, have been told many times to change, and have become accustomed to returning to the practitioner with an inbuilt sense of failure and sometimes resentment. Many see their visits to the practitioner as a ritual in which they have to endure some admonishment before they can begin to express their own agenda. They are reminded of their failures. This harms their sense of self-efficacy and undermines their sense of themselves as people who can make things happen, as opposed to being at the mercy of urges and stresses. However, just as failure often begets failure, nothing breeds success like success; success more or less ensures that the patient will be able to come back next time with good news, and this may be the first step in a new way of viewing themselves and the practitioner–patient relationship. Goals like agreeing not to increase the number of cigarettes smoked or taking the dog for a walk around the block twice a week can be the first small steps down a long road to healthier living.

Resistance will often rear its head:

Well, I would love to give up smoking, I really would, but each time I try, I just about bite the kids' heads off. Even my husband says, *For God's sake, go and have a cigarette if this is what giving up does to you.*

The thoughtless response is to say:

I'm not going to collude with that. Of course giving up is tough. But after biting on the bullet for a week or two, you'll get over it. Sometimes in life, you've just got to stop making excuses and get down to business.

Such an approach is likely to damage the practitioner—patient relationship and may even result in the patient changing practitioners or not consulting when it would be appropriate to do so. An alternative approach is agreeing with those aspects of the patient's comments that are accurate and then to shift focus:

I know. For some people, giving up smoking can play havoc with their nerves. It really can be tough. I've seen people climb the walls, and I'm sorry that nicotine withdrawal affects you that way. But these days, there are treatments for that craving. They don't take it away, but they help take the edge off it. What do you know about nicotine replacement therapy, for example, you know, the gum or the patches? And there's other stuff too now.

This may also be met with further resistance:

Well, I've tried the patches and they don't work for me.
It's too expensive.
My friend had terrible mouth ulcers when he started on the gum. I don't fancy that.

Sometimes it seems that whatever the practitioner says will be countered by *Yes, but* in one form or another. This is a signal to avoid entering into a head-banging interaction where the smoker and practitioner *Yes, but* each other in a series of sterile encounters. Rather, move to closure, summarize and emphasize personal choice or control as a good way of ending:

Sure. You get serious withdrawal symptoms and you have problems with nicotine replacement therapy. And at the same time, giving up smoking remains the single most important thing you could do to improve your health now and to live a longer life. As you said earlier, that's important for you and your family. I agree 100% that there are no easy ways to give up smoking. At the end of the day, it's your life, and you have got to make some tough decisions for yourself. Nicotine replacement was just one suggestion. Maybe you could come up with a few of your own that might be better suited to your needs. After all, you are expert in what you want from life and what will or will not work for you when it comes to quitting smoking. I'll be around if you want to talk about ideas that you come up with at any time.

KEY POINT

Smokers are already feeling judged and defensive before you raise the issue. You will need to work really hard to show empathy. Genuine (not appalled) curiosity about what they like about smoking and why they are reluctant to give up will help to create rapport.

CARDIAC REHABILITATION: LOTS TO DISCUSS
TYPICAL SCENARIO

You are a cardiac rehabilitation specialist nurse. A patient attends after a diagnosis of stable angina. She drinks 35 units a week, is overweight, does very little exercise, smokes, and regularly eats fast or fried foods.

GOALS

- To establish and maintain rapport with the patient. Change and its maintenance are likely to make up a lifelong process and the patient will benefit from a trusting, supportive, and understanding relationship with a practitioner.
- For the practitioner to accept that small shifts in attitude or taking a new look at an old problem is a worthy beginning.
- To promote an appropriate level of concern about risk (the patient should ideally be neither blasé nor so worried as to be incapacitated by anxiety).
- To promote self-efficacy and responsibility.
- To view lifestyle holistically in that each aspect usually affects another; changing one unhealthy behavior may lead to change with another. However, keep the focus on practicalities rather than making global exhortations for dramatic sea changes in personality and behavior.
- To avoid increasing resistance.

PRINCIPLES AND STRATEGIES

- Do not give the same talk to everyone. Target your information to the needs of the patient. Each one is a unique human being with unique challenges, fears, and hopes, and each deserves your full attention and understanding. Establish what the patient already knows about the causes and course of his or her condition.
- Share information in language appropriate to the patient in a nonjudgmental and nonthreatening way.
- Sensitively raise the issue of lifestyle change.
- Use an agenda-setting chart to identify the patient's main current concerns and readiness to address each behavior.
- Assess importance and confidence for change when focusing on a single behavior.
- Typical Day strategy.
- Pros and cons.
- Brainstorming solutions.
- Negotiate attainable goals.

POSSIBLE PRACTICE

Practitioner: I'm pleased you're feeling a bit better, and getting on OK with the tablets. But before we go on any further, I just want to say that the most important factor in your recovery, even more than taking the pills, will be how well you look after yourself, your lifestyle. This depends on what you know about [your condition]. So I'd like to begin by checking what your information needs are, I want to check with you on your understanding of your condition.

Patient: Well, from what I gather, I've got a touch of angina. Stable angina. Nothing too serious, or so I have been told, so long as I continue with the tablets and don't push myself too hard.

Practitioner: Do you know what causes angina? What is happening inside your body, do you think?

Patient: It's a shortage of blood to the heart, or so they say. The heart is starved of oxygen a bit. Furring up of the arteries that take the blood to the heart muscle, or something, by cholesterol. But the tablets will lower the cholesterol so…needn't be too bad.

Notice the resistance emerging already (the patient is minimizing), and notice too that the patient's level of anxiety about her condition, on the surface at any rate, is perhaps inappropriately low. Try a simple reflective listening statement; these are statements (not questions) which reflect the meaning of what the patient has just said. The practitioner's tone goes down at the end of the sentence. Such statements invite an explanatory response from the patient.

Practitioner: Your angina, it's not too serious then.

Patient: Well, lots of people have it, and I guess some do go on to have heart attacks. But mine is mild and the tablets will remove the cause.

Another reflective listening statement could be used at this point: *You might or might not have a heart attack yourself.* Or the practitioner could move to a direct question.

Practitioner: What do you understand of the causes of the problem? What could turn your mild angina into a very serious heart attack even if you are taking tablets?

Patient: Well, they blame everything on smoking and they told me in the hospital that the smoking and the cholesterol brought this on and could make it worse. But I don't smoke any more than most of my friends.

Avoid this invitation to get into a resistance-enhancing argument by responding in a challenging way to this tantalizing but dangerous bait. *Roll with the resistance.* Try agreement and a shift in focus to increase this patient's anxiety to an appropriate level.

Practitioner: You are 100% right! Angina is caused by the heart muscle being starved of oxygen by narrowed blood vessels, and smoking and cholesterol make it worse. Smoking is by far the most important thing that affects your condition right now. But it can also be made worse by being overweight, drinking too much, stress, and not exercising. You are also right that your angina is mild at the moment. But there is nevertheless damage to your arteries, and it could get a lot more serious quite quickly. Changing some of the aspects of your life that lead to narrowing of the arteries could help you live a much longer, pain-free, and active life.

Patient: Yeah. But right now it's mild and under control.

> This patient continues to deny the seriousness of her problem. Amplified reflection is a strategy that could be tried here. The goal is to reflect back to the patient in an amplified or exaggerated form. This should be done very carefully, avoiding sarcasm or hostility.

Practitioner: So, you should be able to get away without changing your lifestyle.

Patient: No, of course not! I really do want to stay healthy. I've got my job and family to think about. [A bit of change talk has at last emerged]

Practitioner: [Emphasizing personal control] Well, you're the one in the driving seat here. It's your life. My job is to give you the information you need to help you make decisions which you feel are best for you and to provide support and help when you decide to change. I'm also concerned about you as one of my patients and as a human being with a condition that could become even more serious quite quickly.

Patient: Yeah, I know you're only trying to help, but I don't want anyone to nag me. The doctor who was in charge of my case when I was admitted in the hospital treated me like I was a naughty schoolgirl.

Practitioner: No nagging, I promise. I know it's useless me trying to make decisions for you and unfortunately neither of us is a schoolgirl anymore! So, I'm going to try something different now. Here is a chart [practitioner produces agenda-setting chart] that may help you in the process of thinking about aspects of your life that have a bad effect on your heart and which can improve your outlook if you change them. But notice here and here are some blank circles for you to put your own concerns into. Concerns that you may feel affect your health or which you just want to talk about. Which of these things, if any, do you feel ready to explore a bit further today?

Patient: Well, I would like to do something about the way I eat. To be honest, that's what really worries me the most. Whatever I say, I hate being fat. [Another piece of change talk]

Practitioner: OK, regarding the food issue, I'm going to ask you two specific questions that involve you rating yourself on a scale of 1–10. How important do you feel healthier eating is to you right now? If 1 is "not at all important" and 10 is "very important," what number would you give yourself right now?

Patient: 9 or 10. Not only for my heart but also for my figure. Sometimes I feel I look like a slob. I deal with the public at work. I don't think looking like a slob helps me professionally.

Practitioner: How confident are you, again on a scale of 1–10, that you could make lasting changes to the way you eat? If 1 is "not at all confident" and 10 is "very confident," what would you give yourself right now?

Patient: Well, 1 work while my partner does all the shopping and cooking. My partner is as thin as a beanpole regardless of what he eats, and he loves his food fried. Don't you just hate the type?

Practitioner: OK, so let's consider ways in which you could tackle this problem and get to eat more of what you would like to. What ideas have you got?

Patient: Well, I could kick him out. No, seriously, perhaps you could talk to him.

Practitioner: Sure, having a meeting with the three of us is one excellent way forward. Any other specific changes you could think of?

Patient: Well, I guess I could do the shopping and cooking if he could pick the kids up from school; that way, I would be more in control of what we eat. But he would have to agree with that.

Practitioner: And how would you eat differently if you could get control of the shopping and cooking?

Patient: I could grill more; go for things like baked potatoes every now and then, more fish. My friend is a vegetarian and she comes up with some pretty good dishes without any meat at all. I quite enjoy being with her when she cooks.

Practitioner: Great. I can see you have some excellent ideas. So why don't we leave it there for now, and you can talk to your partner about the question of what you eat and how it could seriously affect what happens to your health. I'd be happy to meet with the two of you, if he feels that would help. I agree that serious change probably involves getting his help. And you will talk about him picking up the kids in exchange for you doing the shopping and cooking. How does that sound?

The ongoing process of monitoring resistance and readiness is crucial in such consultations; patients are coming to terms with the loss of aspects of their health, and adjustment is a complex and dynamic process. Different people will use varying strategies to deal with it, and the same person may change quite quickly in terms of how he or she reacts to bad news. In the foregoing scenario, the patient's defense was to minimize the problem. However, some patients will feel like they have received a death sentence and are frightened to embark on certain changes (e.g., exercising or having sex after a heart attack). Other patients will argue that there is no point in change because their condition is beyond palliation. So, while the goal was to raise the level of anxiety in the above scenario, sharing information will be important to reduce anxiety in other patients who are too anxious to take practical steps for change.

KEY POINT

The trickiest bit is to allow the patient time to come to terms with the diagnosis while getting some lifestyle changes made as soon as possible to minimize risk and harm. Being sensitive to resistance and picking up on change talk are the ways to monitor how fast the process can proceed.

ENCOURAGING SAFER SEXUAL BEHAVIORS
TYPICAL SCENARIOS

You are a nurse working in a family planning clinic. Your next patient says, *I've got a regular partner now and I'd like to be on the pill.*

You are a doctor in a genitourinary medicine clinic. A patient asks you about a rash on his penis. He tells you he is gay.

GOALS

- To develop a trusting relationship where frank discussion about sensitive issues is comfortable.
- To maintain reasonable boundaries and avoid excessive intimacy.
- To enhance knowledge of safe sex and promote low-risk sexual behavior.
- To enhance the patient's sense of being in control and of being able to say "no" in an uncomfortable situation.

PRINCIPLES AND STRATEGIES

- Establish good enough rapport to be able to raise health promotion issues sensitively.
- Establish the patient's information needs.
- Avoid giving a hurried, uncomfortable lecture.
- Assess importance and enhance confidence to practice safe sex.
- Use scaling questions.
- Try eliciting the pros and cons of an aspect of the practice of safe sex.

POSSIBLE PRACTICE

Practitioner: Sure, I'm happy to help find the best contraception for you and also be a resource for you on sexual health more generally. I appreciate the fact that you have taken this responsible step to come and talk about it all. We'll go through the more medical aspects of your choices, including the pill, in a minute, but would you mind if we first discussed some of the wider implications of being sexually active first? To save me gabbling on about things you already know, can I ask you to tell me a bit about what being sexually active means to you as a person?

Patient: It's kind of a bit awkward talking to you about how I feel. But I guess I do feel I'm ready for it now, and it's something I want to be able to do. But I do get a bit worried. Well, Mark wanted me to go on the pill…he doesn't always like using condoms and sometimes we just don't. I get worried…and they are such a hassle.

Practitioner: Could we spend a moment talking a bit about condoms? Using condoms is crucial to the practice of safe sex, especially if you are not in a long-established relationship. How important is using condoms to you right now? I'm going to be quite specific and ask you to rate its importance to you on a scale of 1−10. If 1 is "not at all important" and 10 is "very important," what number would you give yourself right now?

Patient: Well, I don't want to catch anything bad. I'm young and want to stay healthy, so I'd give myself a 9.

Practitioner: OK. Now how confident are you that you could practice safe sex every time you make love? Again, if 1 is "not at all confident" and 10 is "very confident," what number would you give yourself right now?

Patient: Perhaps a 5 or 6. Mark doesn't like to use them, and I'm not wild about them either. Mark sometimes seems to think I don't trust him if I ask him to put on a condom. Nothing bad has happened yet.

Practitioner: So, you would like to use condoms all the time but it's not always easy to do. What would help you to move from a 5 to a 10, and practice safe sex every time you made love?

Patient: It's Mark, I guess. I find it difficult to insist sometimes. I'd need him to be more supportive.

Conversely, the practitioner could leave out the numbers and ask the importance and confidence questions in his or her own style:

How important do you feel using condoms is for you in your life right now?

How confident are you in your present situation that you could make sure you always had condom-protected sex?

Returning to the problem of the patient asserting her views with her partner:

Practitioner: Do you think you could talk to him about it at a time when you are not about to make love?

Patient: Well, it is difficult. But if there is something on the television about sex, perhaps we could talk then.

Practitioner: Do you want to run through with me the kinds of things you would say as a kind of rehearsal? So when you do raise it, you've got all you want to say in your mind.

Patient: Well, I want to tell him that I want to use condoms not because I don't trust him, but because it's something that everyone should be doing. I heard a talk about it. Stamping out AIDS and keeping my chances open for having a baby later.

Practitioner: Great! As you say, it's something all people in your situation should be doing. Now, let's get on to the pill itself. If you were to start the pill, what do you think about using both a condom and the pill early on in relationships?

This patient had a high importance score and a lower confidence score. Using pros and cons might have worked with someone to whom practicing safe sex was less important. For example,

Practitioner: You gave yourself only a 2 or 3 for importance to you of using condoms. Perhaps you could tell me what you dislike about using condoms and then say what you think is good about using condoms every time you have sex?

Patient: I don't like using them because I feel sex is less natural, the sensation is, you know, less, especially for the man, and I don't want to upset him or spoil it for him, and asking your partner to put on a condom can spoil the moment, like taking a cold shower, or so he says!

Practitioner: OK, tell me what might be good about using condoms?

Patient: Well, I know that it might cut down my chances of getting AIDS and other infections. But that's it.

Practitioner: So, on the one hand, it's more natural without a condom, and putting one on can spoil the magic of sex, your partner doesn't like using them at all and it's not always easy to ask him to put one on. On the other hand, using a condom could save you from getting infected with the HIV virus and getting other diseases like gonorrhea. So, where does that leave you in your thinking about using condoms now?

Resistance may take many forms. Most people underestimate their risk of being infected compared with their understanding of the risks to others.

Practitioner: Can I just check back with you on one thing? What do you know about the risks of unsafe sex? What are your chances of getting infected with sexually transmitted infections including HIV?

Patient: Nothing has happened yet and why should it? I don't sleep around and neither does Mark. We trust each other.

The practitioner may try simple reflection. This is best done in the form of a simple statement.

Practitioner: You're not worried about getting a sexually transmitted infection.

Patient: I'm not saying that. Of course I'm worried about getting an infection. Only a fool would not be worried about it. I saw a program on, what is it, chlamydia? And the HPV vaccine? [Change talk begins to flow]

KEY POINT

Changing sexual behavior is complex. Even practical matters can have huge emotional significance, both to the individual and to the relationship. Reflective listening is a key skill in helping emotionally laden consultations to flow.

WEIGHT MANAGEMENT

Losing weight is not a behavior; it's the result of behaviors! At the conceptual level, losing weight is a simple matter. Being overweight is the result of an imbalance, too many calories in and not enough out. Either eat less or differently, or exercise more, or both. Also, eating less or differently is likely to reduce weight more than increasing exercise, although the two are synergistic; while one is exercising, one generally does not feel like eating! Crash diets seldom result in long-term weight reduction; small, feasible changes to one's overall lifestyle applied consistently over time will have the best chance of long-term benefit. What could be simpler? The plethora of wonder diets and the rapidly increasing obesity epidemic demonstrate that nothing could be more complicated. Being overweight is the end result of complex forces that range from individual understanding and motivation to cultural factors, economics, transport, and town planning. It goes to the very fabric of how society organizes itself. So, individual behaviors have to be seen in the broadest of contexts. This is not to say that there is no point in engaging with individuals about weight. Quite the contrary: appropriate engagement can steer individuals to a path of feasible, sustainable healthier eating and exercise, and change in one family member will influence the whole family unit, modeling future behavior for children, the most vulnerable to premature disease and death from obesity and a sedentary lifestyle.

TYPICAL SCENARIO

You are a nurse doing well-child checks in a community clinic. You weigh an obviously overweight child and notice he is above the 95th percentile for weight. His mother is also obviously in the obese category. The mother seems unconcerned about her own and her child's weight and does not react when you mention the child's weight. She is not asking you for help.

GOALS

- To raise the subject and engage with the mother without causing her to "turn her back" on you.
- To avoid individual blame while prompting the value of individual behavior change.
- To recognize the cultural and environmental contributions to the problem.
- To ensure that you do not jump ahead of the patient by assuming that they recognize the problem!
- To promote an understanding that small changes sustained over time will have large effects.
- To come to owned decisions based on a clear understanding of the risks of not changing, and what is feasible and sustainable for the patient, child, and family.
- To promote a "whole-family" approach; change in one individual family member alone will not solve this family's behavior.

PRINCIPLES AND STRATEGIES

- To establish rapport and obtain permission to discuss the subject without making the mother feel judged, threatened, or defensive.
- The Typical Day strategy may help to establish rapport, help you understand the patient's lifestyle and give you a window into how eating and exercise do (or do not) fit into their lives.
- Pros and cons can be used if there is little importance attached to the idea of change.
- Given that being overweight is the end result of a number of complex behaviors, use an agenda-setting process (with the aid of a chart or purely verbally) to ensure a good understanding of the complexity of the causes and to put the mother in the driving seat of both the decision-making process and in implementing solutions outside the consultation.
- Assess importance and enhance confidence concerning specific areas of focus (e.g., more exercise).

POSSIBLE PRACTICE

Practitioner: OK, so as you can see, Taylor is here on the chart. That means that he is heavier than 95%, no in fact 97%, of boys his age. What's your view on how he's doing, weight wise?

Mother: Well, we are all a little big in our family. Taylor is no different. We are just pretty big people.

One approach here would be to challenge this statement and engage into an argument with the mother. However, this is likely to result in a rather sterile discussion about who is right and who is wrong and may increase resistance to tackling this problem and to future engagement with the health service on this issue. Another approach would be to agree with her, as there is an element of truth in what she says. Then shift focus.

Practitioner: Sure. You are right. Some families are just bigger. But when children get to Taylor's weight, this can start causing quite serious problems. What's your understanding of how Taylor's weight will affect his happiness and health, especially as he gets older?

Mother: Well, I guess I have heard about the diabetes thing. My husband has got, what did they call it, "impaired glucose tolerance" or something?

Practitioner: Yes, and diabetes as you know can be pretty serious. Would you like more information about this kind of thing? No? You get an earful each time you turn on the TV? Your aunt had it too? Well then, I just wondered if we could spend a few minutes quickly talking about eating and activity in your family? It would help me understand things better from your perspective, and maybe together we can consider one or two small changes that could make an important difference for all of your health? OK? So, to help me with this, maybe think of a typical day in your family, like say Tuesday if that was reasonably typical for you guys.

Begin with when you all woke up and take me through the day, telling me about how eating, food, and any exercise and activity, or even any potential opportunity for exercise, fits in.

Mother: Well, it's a pretty busy household I can tell you, and we don't get much time for fancy cooking if that's what you're thinking about. From the time the alarm goes off, it's "go go go," getting them breakfast and off to school. The older kids usually get their own breakfast. They usually make a sandwich with whatever is in the fridge. Chocolate spread is their favorite. I give Taylor the same usually too or if I don't get time, he has chocolate or chips on the way to school. I hate the idea of them being hungry at school. They get their lunch at school. I once tried making them all packed lunches, I know that they could be healthier, but there isn't time. Then it's in the car and the school run, well it feels like a run to me…

Practitioner: OK. Now what we do know is that any one single diet course might help one person for a little while, but changes in the way the whole family approaches this is likely to help improve the whole family's health most. So, let's consider some of the things that influence weight. There is exercise, you know, which not only includes sport and running and so on. It's also walking to school, taking the stairs instead of the escalator, and stuff like that. Walking the dog. Then there is eating: the amount you eat, you know portion sizes, snacking and things like that, and then also the type of food. Fried and high-fat foods versus the healthier stuff: vegetables, fruit, cereal, and so on. Does this make any sense? What's your understanding of healthier living here?

Mother: Well, I know what you mean. I know the chocolates on the way to school and usually a can of soda, if I'm honest, don't do him much good. And I wish, one day, I could get to the point where we take our own lunches to school and work. Some fruit as well.

Practitioner: Yes and possibly cereal rather than chocolate sandwiches for breakfast? Do they ever get involved in cooking with you?… OK so we've chatted about food for a while. What about activity? Are there any changes, no matter how small, in things you do every day that could help here?

Mother: It's the school that makes me feel guilty. I always take the car, and the traffic and the parking is terrible. Truth be told, it takes me just as long as walking, and with the kids yelling in the car, it's a nightmare trip. I hate it…

Notice that the potential solutions are coming from the mother. They are "whole-family" focused, and there is an absence of criticism, threat, and judgment in this discourse. Now perhaps is the time to find out what changes the mother feels able to work on in the short term and to negotiate some form of follow-up.

Practitioner: So, excellent. You've come up with some very practical and workable ideas for changing that could improve the health of the whole family. We've spoken about changes you could make about food and eating. You've also mentioned a great possibility about building in more activity into the day. Now it's decision time. Which, if any, of these changes do you feel you are ready to tackle right now?... Before you go, though, can I ask you what the biggest challenge will be for you to implement these changes? Getting the kids used to it? Just as I thought. Now let's talk that through quickly... OK. Well, that's a pretty impressive plan. How about we meet in 1 month? I will check Taylor over again and we can chat about your family's progress.

KEY POINT

Weight is a very personal issue but influenced by many contextual factors. Raising the subject, especially with people who are not asking for help about weight, is a delicate matter. Well-intentioned but inappropriately directive approaches can cause considerable harm. Elicit solutions from key decision-makers in the family that are feasible for all to implement and follow. Focus on the system rather than any one individual. Small changes implemented consistently will bring large benefit for all.

WHEN THE PROBLEM IS MOOD, NOT BEHAVIOR
TYPICAL SCENARIO

You are consulting with a woman who has three school-aged children. She tells you that she feels terrible and that she is not coping very well. Life seems just one big struggle. You know that improved mood often flows from the sufferer changing aspects of his or her everyday life, so recovery and behavior change are usually closely linked.

GOALS

- To provide safe care, offering appropriate treatments that may involve other practitioners. However, use your interaction to promote a sense of self-worth, hope, and control over at least some aspects of the world.
- To be supportive and empathetic, without colluding with defeatism.
- To negotiate goals that are more or less certain to be attained; assert the value of seemingly small achievements.
- To promote a shorter-term, day-by-day view of the process of recovery rather than setting daunting long-term goals.
- To ensure that expectations for recovery are realistic. The patient should expect slow progress as well as setbacks.

PRINCIPLES AND STRATEGIES

- Typical Day strategy.
- Invite the patient to reflect on his or her daily achievements.
- Use a modified agenda-setting chart.

- Assess importance and confidence for embarking on an alternative, control-enhancing strategy.
- Brainstorm solutions.
- Negotiate short-term, attainable goals.

POSSIBLE PRACTICE

Where new therapeutic behaviors have not yet been identified by either party in the consultation, beginning with assessing importance and confidence to change is inappropriate. The Typical Day strategy is a better place to start because it builds rapport, increases the practitioner's insight into the patient's life, and provides a direct route into physical symptoms, psychological state, and the contextual modifying factors. This biopsychosocial approach to diagnosis and treatment is especially important in patients with a mood disorder:

> I wonder if I could ask you to tell me a little more about your life right now and the problems you are facing? It would help me to understand the situation better if you could pick a typical day in your life, say like yesterday, for example, and take me through it from when you woke up. Tell me about the things you struggled with and how you felt at the time.

The patient may need further encouragement and brief prompting to give the practitioner a picture of her day, the problems that arose, and her feelings at each hurdle. As the story unfolds, it is likely that the practitioner will gain an in-depth knowledge of the patient's level of function, variation in mood states throughout the day, view of the future, existing coping strategies, support base, and contributing external factors to the low mood. Assessments of danger to self in this way (possibility of deliberate self-harm) may be more sensitive than traditional direct questioning, as an account of a typical day will provide a more accurate assessment of the frequency and intrusiveness of such thoughts.

The practitioner is often left with a genuine sense of the enormous effort that a patient in such a position is making to get through each day. Several important achievements in this day's struggle are likely to emerge, which the patient could rightly feel proud of. The practitioner may simply ask the patient to identify and then reflect on such apparently small achievements:

> Great. Now, I really can see what you mean when you say that life is a huge struggle for you at the moment. I can see that there are some things that you have handled in a way that frustrates you. But I must say, given how you are feeling, there are things you told me that I, for one, was deeply impressed by. Perhaps you could list the things that you realize you handled well...
>
> That's excellent! When one is feeling low, it's common not to be able to identify anything positive about oneself, and forcing yourself to list not only the negative but also the positive things, no matter how apparently trivial they might seem, is an important discipline to nurture as one begins a journey down the road to feeling better. At the end of each day, listing such achievements, no matter how small, may help to get the day in better perspective. I have to say that given how bad you are feeling, I am deeply moved by how hard you are trying to keep things going and how much you are

succeeding in achieving. I know you are very irritable; your shouting at the kids worries you and sometimes you feel you just can't go on. But somehow you do carry on and are there for them. You put them to bed, read a story to the little guy, kissed them, and told them you loved them. As you say, the fact that you get three kids off to school each day and are there for them when they come back, you feed them, you give them care, attention and love, and you get them to bed are significant achievements. One just has to go through a day like that once to know how exhausting it can be.

Now let's tackle the more frustrating things that you mentioned. I am going to draw a few circles on this blank page and I'll write each frustration that you mentioned in a circle. We call this thing an agenda-setting chart. OK, so here we've got poor sleep, here screaming at the kids, here housework, not doing anything to relax, and finally smoking too much. I want you to select one of these to work on in the next while. Try to choose something that you feel reasonably able to tackle right now… Whew! That's brave! Screaming at the kids in the morning! That is a serious problem at a time when I know you are feeling at your worst and at your most helpless.

Assess importance and confidence in change. Importance is likely to be high and confidence low:

You mentioned that not shouting at the kids in the mornings is very important to you but you are not confident you can manage to change. OK, so what ideas do you have for improving this aspect of your day?… Great. As you say, you could get up a bit earlier, be a bit more organized, have a better routine, and prepare things a bit more before they come down and, as you say, you could explain to them the night before that things are difficult for you. Some day, you might give them each a specific task to help get the day going smoothly. That will take a while, I agree, to get them into the routine and to know you mean business, but if you could pull it off somewhere down the line, that would be a major achievement. But for the moment, why don't we begin with you setting a timetable for the morning, waking up 15 min earlier and getting things ready before they come down? That way, when they are there, you might feel more relaxed and in control.

Say the patient chose to build some quality relaxation time into her day. The practitioner might not even assess importance and confidence because he or she may already have a good feel for these two domains:

So, the time in the middle of the day that right now you spend on your own when you feel worst, when thoughts of all the problems come flooding into your mind. Is there anything active you can think of that you might enjoy doing during this time?… Going for a walk if the weather is fine, seeing a friend, taking in a movie, spoiling yourself at the shops; sure, all good suggestions… Is there a goal that you would like to set for yourself in this regard?… Great! Why don't we say that for at least 1 day this week, you might go out for a walk in the middle of the day?

Summarizing is important both to ensure a common understanding of the goals and to ensure that there is agreement about what is expected.

Practitioner: Excellent. So to summarize, at the end of each day, as I understand it, you have agreed to make a deliberate effort to routinely consider the things you did OK and well, and not to think about just the things that disappoint you. It might even be a good idea to write your positive achievements down in list form at the end of each day. Second, you are going to try to get up a little earlier to prepare for the kids so that you can feel more in control when they come down (and 1 day in the week, you might go out for a walk on your own in the middle of the day). Is that how you see what we agreed? Do you feel these goals are manageable?

Patient: [Putting her head in her hands] All this is easy for you to say. I'm the one who has to do it.

> This resistance may take the practitioner slightly by surprise and would not have become apparent had the practitioner not checked back with the patient. The unthinking response is to say, *Listen, all I'm trying to do is to help you make a program to enable you to help yourself. You have to get moving on this one!* This may make the patient feel badgered and even more defeated. When response to goals is less than enthusiastic, it could be that importance and confidence have been misjudged and it is worth checking back. In this case, confidence is clearly the main issue.

Practitioner: I know that life is tough for you right now. Perhaps I have underestimated exactly how difficult it is for you to make changes right now. How confident are you that you could make a list each day of your achievements and get up 15 min earlier to get ready for the kids?

Patient: I don't know. It takes me so long to get to sleep. I do my best sleeping at the end, you know, just before I wake. The thought of getting up earlier just makes me feel sick, even though I know it might help with the kids.

Practitioner: That's fine. Keeping the list, how confident are you that you could do that?

Patient: The list I think I could manage.

Practitioner: Good. The important thing is that you make a start, and I feel that keeping a list of all your achievements each day is an excellent beginning. Will you show it to me when we meet again?

> End with a supportive statement and a note of realistic optimism.

Practitioner: Now, just before we part, I want to say that it has taken a while to get to feel so bad. Getting to where you would like to be will not be easy and you will have many setbacks along the way. But by focusing on small things and looking at the next step rather than the whole journey, I'm confident that things will gradually improve. Doubtless, there will be some days on which you feel back at square one, but as time goes by, these episodes generally last a shorter and shorter time for people who are beginning to take control of their low mood. So, let's meet up next week and you can let me know how you got on with the goal you set today.

> The content of the goals is less important than ensuring that there is some sense of achievement built into the next meeting. The crucial switch is for this patient to develop a sense of herself as someone who can, to some extent at least, control her situation, rather than seeing herself as simply reacting to events.

KEY POINT

Self-efficacy is the key focus here, and finding small manageable steps is the way to build it. Ensure that you check all along what feels manageable to the patient. People with low mood can feel overwhelmed by tasks that would not worry them at all in another state of mind.

PATIENTS WHO DO NOT HELP THEMSELVES

Many practitioners will recognize elements of the following scenarios in their clinical practice. While not specifically dealing with each scenario, what follows should generate some ideas that are relevant to all similar situations.

TYPICAL SCENARIOS

You are working in an outpatient clinic for people with epilepsy. A patient with frequent seizures swears he or she is taking the medication as prescribed. Blood levels of the drug are erratic. You increase the dose of his or her drug. The blood levels come back low. The patient says, *I can't understand why my blood level is so low because I take my medicine as regular as clockwork, every night before I go to bed.*

You are a nurse in a clinic for people with diabetes. A patient with diabetes insists he or she is taking his or her medicine as prescribed and is sticking to his or her diet. When he or she arrives for blood tests, the random sugar (one measure of short-term adherence) is always very low but the glycosylated hemoglobin (testing longer-term blood sugar levels) is very high. This suggests he or she takes his or her medicines only for those few days just before seeing you.

You are a nurse running a chronic disease management clinic for people with hypertension. A patient with hypertension attends faithfully, but despite numerous medication changes and additions, his or her blood pressure has not changed. It did come down while he or she was in the hospital receiving supervised treatment. The patient says, *Blood pressure still up? Are you sure the doctor has prescribed the right medication?*

You are a general medical practitioner in a busy practice. The mother of a child with bad eczema wants you to prescribe a stronger steroid cream. She insists she is using oils in the bath and moisturizing creams all the time. However, these were last prescribed over 8 months ago, and if used properly, they would have run out in a month.

GOALS

- To be honest without alienating the patient or provoking resistance. Fighting with these people would achieve nothing!
- To avoid being judgmental.
- To understand what medication means to patients in practical terms (the hassle of using medication as prescribed) and in terms of their views of themselves (e.g., stigma).
- To be flexible and to negotiate. Patients have to make their own appraisals of risk and benefit and live with the consequences. Practitioners cannot take medicine

for patients. The practitioner's job is to provide the structure and information for patients to make choices that are best for them.
- To make the treatment experience as user-friendly as possible.

PRINCIPLES AND STRATEGIES

- Raise the subject in an honest yet nonconfrontational way; explain your confusion or the apparent contradictions in what you are told and what you find.
- Speak initially in general terms before putting the patient personally on the spot.
- Assess the importance to the patient of taking the medicines as prescribed.
- Promote the patient's confidence in his or her ability to take the medicine as prescribed.
- Use scaling questions with a view to increasing importance and building confidence.
- Check the patient's understanding of what is expected and how he or she is actually taking the medicine. The Typical Day strategy may be useful.
- If the problem is one of low personal importance, provide information in a nonjudgmental way for the patient to factor into his or her decision-making. The pros and cons strategy may be useful. If the problem is mainly confidence in implementing a decision to take the medicines, then brainstorm solutions.
- Negotiate attainable goals that are acceptable to both patient and practitioner.

POSSIBLE PRACTICE

Gary, I'm glad that you are feeling so well. I just want to be sure I know exactly when and what medicines you are using. Would you mind if we just spent a moment or two focusing on other aspects of the medication? Can I just ask you how important taking the medicine is to you right now? So that I can get a really accurate sense of what you feel, if 1 is "not at all important" and 10 is "very important," what number would you give yourself for how important taking the medicine is to you right now?... 5! Excellent.

OK, say you did decide that taking your medicine was very important to you, how confident are you that you could begin and continue to take your medicine as prescribed? If 1 is "not at all confident" and 10 is "100% confident" that you could stick to the regime exactly, what number would you give yourself right now?... 5 as well.

Let me ask you now, for importance of taking the medicine to you, you gave yourself a 5. Why not a 1?

I see, you feel medicine might help you in the long term, but what happens to you right now is more important. And right now the medicine makes you feel sick.

Right. You also gave yourself a 5 for confidence in your ability to take the medicine as prescribed. What would help you to move up from a 5 to say a 7 or 8?

Here, the patient may identify practical barriers in his or her daily life (e.g., inconvenience; taking inhalers while at work) and psychological barriers (e.g., stigma, a teenager with diabetes feeling like an outsider when not able to drink a lot of alcohol with friends).

If little emerges to work on as a result of assessing importance and confidence, try the Typical Day strategy:

Taking any sort of medication every day is tedious in anyone's language. There are very few people who like taking medicine, and yet it is an important part of controlling illness. And people are all different in how taking medicine affects them and how they feel about it. It would help me to give the best input into your care if you would give me a clearer picture of how you feel about your medicine and how it fits into your life. A good way into this would be if you would think of a recent typical day in your life and take me through it, telling me when you use medicines and how you feel about it at the time. Take me through yesterday, for example.

During this process, ask patients how they feel about themselves and the medicines. Fascinating insights commonly emerge. Taking medicines is often inconvenient and causes unpleasant side effects in ways the practitioner never imagined. It may also remind the patients of their loss of health, loss of control, and of associated stigma:

Heavens above! With all that going on, it must be difficult to remember to take the medicine exactly as we doctors and nurses expect you to. You've certainly told me a thing or two that I hadn't thought about before, and I am at least beginning to understand what this illness means from your point of view. This can only help me in providing you with the best information tailored to your unique circumstances so that you can make decisions about your own health that are right for you. After all, it's you that has to take (or not take) the medicines and it's you who has to live with the consequences.

This could lead into asking about pros and cons:

OK, fine. You really miss that feeling that you are a normal, healthy human being, just like your friends, and that's especially bad when you go out with them on Saturday nights and when you go down to the beach on the weekend. Is there a way of taking some, if not all, of your medicine that might not interfere with your sense of who you are so much? Give me all your ideas, no matter how wild or crazy they may seem.

Often the practitioner may find that the patient is already taking huge risks in any case, and relatively simple advice and acceptance may diminish overall risk-taking, even if exact compliance is not achieved. At least honesty is injected into the practitioner—patient relationship when suboptimal compliance can be discussed openly:

Patient: You mean you wouldn't mind if I didn't test my sugars on the weekends and vacations, so long as I took a lower dose of my insulin on those days?

Practitioner: What I mind is not the issue here. What matters is how you feel and to get right the balance between your enjoyment of life, control of the illness now, and possible long-term complications. All I am saying is that giving yourself a break may mean that you look after yourself better overall. I'm prepared to support you if you want to give it a try, so long as we regularly reassess the situation. What do you think?

Then negotiate acceptable, attainable goals:

Practitioner: So for the time being, you've decided to give yourself only one shot of long-acting insulin on Saturday mornings before you go out with your friends, and on these days you won't check your sugars. But on other days, you'll stick with your twice-daily dosage as prescribed and also check your sugars. See me in a month and tell me how it goes.

If low importance is the main problem, the pros and cons strategy is useful in bringing the decision dilemma into sharp, conscious focus. Often, compliance issues are pushed into the background of one's mind, and although knowledge may be adequate, a kind of noncompliance by default occurs rather than through a considered, owned decision-making process. Pros and cons may also give the practitioner insights into the patient's information needs.

Arguing and denying are common features of consultations that focus on adherence to prescribed medication. As always, the practitioner should initially turn down the patient's invitation to an immediate boxing match in the consulting room. One way forward is simply explaining one's puzzlement to the patient. Where possible, frame contradictions in terms of generalities rather than in the individual's specific behavior. If possible, put the patient in the role of the problem solver, rather than the practitioner seeing him- or herself as an investigator whose cunning has tripped the patient up:

Well, I don't understand it. You are taking your pills and yet your blood levels are low. Most people on this dose of pills will have a blood level of X. What do you think could be happening?

Gosh! It's 3 months since we last prescribed that inhaler for you. Most people use up those inhalers in half that time. What do you think could be happening to your asthma?

Most children get better using very little of the potentially dangerous steroid cream because they use a lot of the moisturizers on a regular basis. What do you think could be happening with your child?

KEY POINT

It is the patient's decision to take medication. The health practitioner's decisions are whether to prescribe a particular drug and what course of action to recommend. Information exchange can be a useful part of helping patients to make informed decisions about their medication use. Used well, this approach gets away from the situation where the practitioner gets frustrated because the patient would not do what he or she is told, and the patient tries to get away with not doing what he or she is told because he or she never wanted to do it in the first place!

PATIENTS WHO WANT MORE MEDICINE

This is an example where practitioners would prefer not to meet patients' stated needs, largely for clinical reasons.

TYPICAL ACUTE PRESCRIBING SCENARIO

You are a primary care physician. Your patient has a sore throat that is almost certainly caused by a virus:

> Yes, you have told me all that before. I know it's probably a virus. Can I have my antibiotics now please?

TYPICAL LONG-TERM PRESCRIBING SCENARIOS

You work in a pain clinic. You are trying to suggest pain management strategies that do not involve strong compound analgesics:

> That is all very well for you to say, but you don't have to live with the pain. I need my prescription.

You are working in a psychiatry outpatient department and see someone who has been on tranquilizers for many years. You raise the subject of the tranquilizers:

> Of course I would prefer not to take the tranquilizers. I'm not really a "pill person." But I do need them every now and then. Can I have a full month's supply this time? It'll save me having to bother you so often.

GOALS

- To practice ethically by avoiding prescribing medicines which are of dubious biomedical benefit or sometimes overtly harmful.
- To encourage patient empowerment by promoting a sense of responsibility for negotiated decisions.
- To at least sow a seed that there are also nonpharmacological ways of coping with patients' problems.
- To preserve the health practitioner–patient relationship.
- To minimize the practitioner's sense of frustration.
- To ensure that the patient feels listened to, supported, and understood.

PRINCIPLES AND STRATEGIES

- When importance is high and confidence is low, assess importance to the patient of a low drug approach and enhance confidence to change.
- Consider how far it is possible and desirable for the practitioner to meet the patient's request on this occasion.
- Hand over as much control as possible to the patient.
- Elicit reasons that are real for the patient about the merits and otherwise of taking the medicines.

- If importance is low, engage in nonjudgmental information sharing.
- Use pros and cons strategy with ambivalent patients.
- Brainstorm solutions to identify options.
- Set attainable goals.

POSSIBLE PRACTICE: ACUTE MEDICATION

How many times are explanations about the inappropriateness of drugs in specific situations met with a dogged determination to get the drug from the practitioner, sometimes at all costs? Under these conditions, it is tempting for practitioners to grit their teeth and either issue the prescription or become challenging. The former solution usually leaves the practitioner feeling frustrated and nothing really changes for the patient. The second response simply increases the practitioner's blood pressure and provokes resistance in the patient!

Let us explore more creative ways out of this situation, with the help of the example of the woman who wants antibiotics for her throat infection that you feel is unlikely to benefit from antibiotic treatment. First, try to establish the importance of a nonantibiotic approach:

Practitioner: I'm not saying I won't prescribe antibiotics under any circumstances, but I feel this is an important decision and we should take it very seriously together. Everyone has their own views on the topic, and I want to be sure that I properly understand yours. What do you feel about antibiotics?

Patient: Well, I know they work for me when I get like this. I need the antibiotics. That is why I have come all this way to see you.

Assessing confidence in implementing a nonantibiotic approach is probably not worthwhile in the face of the level of importance that the patient attaches to taking antibiotics now. Generally, if the importance of change is very low, always address that before exploring confidence.

Here we have a situation where the patient and practitioner are on opposite ends of the importance spectrum. When it comes to taking antibiotics for this condition, this patient rates importance highly and this practitioner rates it as low. Changing this patient's perception of the importance of antibiotics while preserving the practitioner–patient relationship in a single consultation may not be possible. A more realistic goal is to be sure that the patient understands that the best medical wisdom is clear that taking antibiotics will not help her to get better more quickly and that the antibiotics carry dangers for which she will have to share responsibility. Perhaps then a seed will be sown and next time, perhaps next year, the patient will be prepared to at least consider ways of dealing with these infections which do not involve antibiotics.

One way of approaching this situation is to say:

I understand your concerns and I will give you the antibiotics after 2 days if you are not already getting better. However, I would not be doing my job if I did not first share with you some concerns. The research shows that… What do you make of this research?

If the patient is not ready to engage, the practitioner may wish to honestly state his or her position and move to closure, emphasizing personal choice and responsibility:

Well, research shows that antibiotics will probably do no good in situations like this. They could even do some harm which can occasionally be life-threatening. Do you know of any dangers associated with antibiotics?… Well there are some dangers that you should know about. Minor side effects like upset stomachs and rashes are common, and serious reactions like bone marrow problems and allergies do very occasionally occur. Using antibiotics also makes bugs resistant to them, which could mean that when you really need them for a life-threatening infection, they don't work so well. I will leave a prescription for you at the front desk and, as I say, if after a day or 2 you aren't beginning to get better, you are welcome to come down and pick it up. You don't need to consult, just pick it up.

Some patients will be aware that antibiotics are a mixed blessing and might be more ambivalent. Here, one may try a pros and cons strategy:

You feel that you probably need antibiotics in this situation. Fair enough, you are the expert when it comes to how you feel now and how these drugs have helped you in the past. I wonder, though, have you heard about some of the problems that can be caused by antibiotics? So that we can be sure that I understand your thinking in this regard, perhaps you could quickly tell me some of the reasons why you think antibiotics are appropriate now and some of the reasons why they might not be.

Some patients will feel that it is very important to try alternatives to drug treatment but are worried how they will manage (low in confidence). Exploring the importance of doing without antibiotics is obviously less critical among these people. Practitioners are likely to get more returns for their efforts if they focus on building confidence to cope differently. Suggesting practical strategies will be useful. In the case of the request for antibiotics for sore throats, one might elicit ideas from the patient and then suggest the use of fluids, antipyretics and analgesics if these have not yet been mentioned. Offer to review the patient within a day, or give the patient a prescription for an antibiotic but ask him or her not to take the drug unless symptoms deteriorate.

POSSIBLE PRACTICE: LONG-TERM MEDICATION

In the case of chronic analgesic or benzodiazepine use, one can offer a very slow program of change where the patient is in the driving seat and the practitioner provides ongoing support. The underlying problem is often a chasm between how the two parties in the consultation view solutions. The patient often wants a biomedical, simple solution, whereas the practitioner sees the situation as a chronic problem best addressed through lifestyle adjustment.

Practitioner: Sure, I'll definitely give you your medication, but I just want to ask you a bit more how you feel about using this amount of dihydrocodeine? Right now, how important to you is cutting down on the amount of painkillers you are using? If 1 is "not at all important" and 10 is "very important," what number would you give yourself right now?

OK, and how confident are you that you could cut down if that was your decision? If 1 is "not at all confident" and 10 is "very confident" that you could cut down and keep on with less medicine, what number would you give yourself right now?

You gave yourself 8 for importance to you of cutting down. Why as high as that?

Patient: Well, I don't like taking medicines. I know they are addictive and I would like to be well again, off all the pills.

Practitioner: What would help your confidence in your ability to cut down and move up from a 4 to an 8 or 9?

If the patient is able to come up with suggestions, the process of brainstorming solutions might continue from here. If the patient is not able to come up with many practical suggestions, try using the Typical Day strategy and then move into brainstorming solutions:

Changing established patterns of medication use is never easy, and I applaud your courage in agreeing to experiment with whether you can do with less. I want you to be the main decision-maker here. We will move at your speed, and I will encourage you to go slowly and to expect setbacks. I will be here to support you in the decisions you make. Now let's see, at the moment you are using 10 pills of dihydrocodeine a day. Take me through a typical day in your life, telling me when your pain gets bad and when you use the tablets. I also want you to think about what else you could have done apart from taking the pills.

Good. I think this has been very useful for me. You have helped me understand the intensity of the pain and the courage you are already showing in managing it.

Practitioners who have heard the detail of the daily lives of their patients will seldom fail to be moved by their accounts of chronic pain or anxiety states and can usually make comments like this with absolute sincerity:

What other options do you have, say when the pain gets bad after lunch? [Practitioner listens carefully to patient's suggestions and then may add one or two of his own] Right, so you could take a pill, you could do something about the house to get your mind off it, you could take the dog for a walk around the block, or you could have a hot bath. Which one of these options do you think you could go for over the next month? Great, so you think you could try and go for a short walk after lunch when the pain gets bad instead of taking a pill. Exercise encourages your body to release natural opiates that also help your mood! And exercise, even if it causes some pain, can prevent deterioration. It strengthens the muscles and that takes pressure off your painful bones. How about we set a goal of, say, using 10 pills less (say 290 rather than 300) over the course of the next month and when we meet again, you can tell me how it's been going, walking the dog instead of using a pill on some days after lunch?

Resistance can manifest in almost every conceivable form in these often fraught situations; for example, anger: *I'm fed up with being told I don't need these pills.*

I do, I tell you. I'm the one who has to live with this constant hell every day of my life; splitting: *Doctor X told me I should never be without these pills*; challenging: *You say these pills can do harm. They are the only thing that has ever helped me* and disagreeing: *I would love to be able to cut down on my pills. But there is nothing else that works*, and so on.

The key to dealing with resistance is convincing the patient that you share the same goals, namely to improve the patient's health. You are acting out of concern and commitment to the patient, not vindictiveness. Establishing this can be the springboard to shifting the focus off biomedical cures to considering personal and social components that affect the patient's suffering. Agreement about the seriousness of the patient's symptoms and then shifting focus is one way of concluding such consultations and opening the door to nonpharmacological approaches at the next visit.

Practitioner: Slow down! No one is talking of abandoning you without any medication or indeed in making changes that you are not ready for. All I'm doing is sharing with you research findings that long-term medication like this can cause some harm. Remember, I'm your doctor and I have a duty to inform all patients about the risks of medicines that I prescribe. I'm focusing on this issue not because I want to be nasty. Quite the opposite. I believe we have exactly the same goals here. We are both interested in your living a happier, healthier life. I see my role as helping you to make decisions which are right for you rather than telling you what to do. Now I believe you 100% when you tell me how terrible you feel without your tranquilizers and painkillers. Anyone who experiences those kinds of feelings would want pills that relieved their symptoms. But it also seems that you feel pretty bad sometimes even when you take the medication. Now I'm committed to working with you on this one. I just think you can feel better, with or without pills, if you also focus on other things that are relevant to how you feel. Let's set aside the question of cutting down the pills for the moment then, and talk about some of the things that influence your anxiety, other than pills.

Patient: Get real. I know you just want to take my pills away from me.

Practitioner: [Being honest and reframing the problem] Look, I make no secret of the fact that I am concerned about the medication. But that's not the only thing I am concerned about. I am concerned about how you feel. Pills are only a small part of your life. Looking at pills in relation to you as a whole person in order to help you feel better overall is my goal.

KEY POINT

Both patient and practitioner almost certainly share the same goal, to maintain the patient in a healthy, pain-free state, and to put any health problems right as soon as they appear. Keeping this sense of an alliance can facilitate the information exchange that will help the patient to make a good decision.

PATIENTS WHO ARE SEEKING UNLIKELY EXPLANATIONS OR CURES

TYPICAL SCENARIO

You are a primary care practitioner. You look at the fat file in front of you and sigh. Fifteen years of pain, numerous rounds of expensive and sometimes dangerous investigations. A human being mutilated by surgeons who have cut this and then that organ out of her in a desperate attempt to "do something." But still the pain goes on. Yes, Mrs. Smith again. You know exactly what she will say to you even before you have called her into the consulting room; it has happened so many times before:

I know all the tests are negative, and in the hospital they said I should see a psychiatrist. But I'm telling you, this kind of pain is not in my head. Surely that new scan I've heard about will be able to identify what's gnawing inside me? If only you would help me sort this pain out, I could start living my life again.

GOALS

- To promote acceptance in both the patient and the practitioner that the patient has taken years to get where she is; improvement is likely to occur only slowly.
- Investing a bit of extra time and emotional energy during this visit may cause a shift in attitude to the problem on the part of either or both parties.
- For the practitioner to accept that medicine *cures* very few problems. A worthy goal is to help people accept and make the most of their imperfect situations and to initiate an approach which does not just seek biomedical solutions to discomfort and distress.
- Never leave the patient feeling abandoned. Preserve hope, but keep this realistic and do not mislead the patient. Offer to see the patient regularly at structured intervals.
- To aim toward an acceptance that there is no "magic bullet" that will cure the patient. A quick fix is not in the cards. The next best thing is adjusting goals from finding a cure to maximizing control over the symptoms.

PRINCIPLES AND STRATEGIES

- Try to see this old problem with fresh eyes; we often think we understand our patients and therefore we spend less time exploring beyond the biomedical to include personal and contextual considerations.
- The Typical Day strategy is often a good place to start in situations where new, alternative behaviors are not yet clearly articulated in the minds of either the patient or the practitioner.
- Information exchange.

- Pros and cons of having further tests at this time.
- Importance and confidence of alternatives to further medical tests.
- Watch resistance closely; assess personal control and consider agreement with a shift in focus.
- Keep an open mind; be flexible and negotiate.
- Set attainable goals.

POSSIBLE PRACTICE

Practitioner: Good morning, Mrs. Smith. Good to see you again. How are things going?

Patient: Not very well at all. I really am trying hard not to bother you and sometimes I feel you must be getting fed up with me and my ongoing problems. But I really think it's getting worse and I can't go on like this. This pain consumes my life, and all I want is to be well again. Now I was reading in a magazine about a man who had pain just like me and the doctors had also told him it was all in his head. Then he had a new, enhanced scan and they found out what it was. They caught it just in time. Now I know I've had the usual scan, but it wasn't the new, enhanced scan. What do you think about me having the new, enhanced scan?

Saying "no" to the new, enhanced scan at this stage would be akin to putting on a pair of boxing gloves. Try agreeing to take the request seriously and then shifting the focus.

Practitioner: OK, sure, the enhanced scan is definitely worth thinking about. Anything that could possibly help you live a fuller life deserves careful consideration. I see myself 100% as your advocate when it comes to tests and treatments. By that, I mean it's my role to help you decide what is likely to help you and indeed what could harm your recovery. There are very few tests that do not have side effects and ever more tests can slow down your recovery; people can focus on tests more than on getting better sometimes! So before we make any decision about further tests, I want to be sure I have a complete picture in my mind so I can give you the best possible advice. I want to know about the exact nature of your symptoms and how they affect your life these days. Often, going over it all again in some detail can shed important light on the subject that I may have forgotten about. Who knows, you might give me new clues about the cause of the problems that I hadn't picked up before. It would help me a lot if you would think of a typical day in your life, say yesterday or the day before, and take me through it, beginning when you woke up, and telling me how you feel as you move through the day.

Patient: Well, I've kind of been through this before, and I can tell you right now you are not going to get me to see a psychiatrist.

The patient has created a massive block to engaging with the practitioner and participating in the Typical Day strategy. Agreement and expressing support for the patient in the face of major stumbling blocks can have profound results.

Practitioner: Fine. No problem. Let's agree on that right now then. No psychiatrists! It's very important for me that you understand that I believe this pain is very serious and real. The last thing I want to do is to send you off to yet another doctor. I am committed to the two of us doing our best to coming to grips with this problem together, and I want to assure you that I will stand by you in this process. But I do need your help. Telling me about a typical day in your life will help us make the best plans about your treatment together.

Patient: OK, I guess. Well, as I've said, I wake up with the pain in my abdomen; as I've said, there is also a full feeling and a pressing feeling on my spine, and then the pain builds up and up while I'm dressing, so I take my pills which don't really help and then I go to the toilet which does ease it a bit but I'm never free of it. Then I try and eat something, otherwise my husband nags me. That usually makes it worse but I do it to keep him quiet. Then he goes off to work and leaves me with the pain…

Practitioner: How do you feel at this time?

Patient: Sometimes, when he goes off, I just want to put my head in a pillow and scream… to be honest, sometimes I do. Sometimes I feel that no one understands what I'm going through. How can they?

The practitioner should avoid invitations to be sidetracked into anything else than the patient's account of her journey through a typical day.

Practitioner: What happens next?

The practitioner listens and asks further questions about how the patient feels at key points. Eventually, the practitioner may ask the patient to reflect on the relationship between her pain, its immediate context and her feeling at the time.

Practitioner: Mrs. Smith, what you've told me will be invaluable to the process of decision-making that we are both working on. I'm just wondering, are you able to identify patterns in your pain: for example, times when your pain is worse or better, and what is going on in your life at the time?

If the patient is not forthcoming, the practitioner may throw in an invitation to reflect on the loneliness she feels in her suffering: *Are there any things you could change which might make you feel more understood and less isolated in your pain?* Remember, in situations like this, radical change is not likely after one interaction along these lines. This patient's journey toward a view of the problem that is not focused purely on biomedical solutions and which incorporates acceptance of pain and adapting to life with pain is likely to be long and hard. Planting a seed for looking at the problem as one of adaptation rather than cure is perhaps the most realistic goal of this consultation.

Practitioner: OK, excellent, well that is a start and I am sure that you might come up with further ideas later. But now I want to turn back to the question of the new, enhanced scan. Why don't we quickly make a list of all the tests you've had, all the specialists you've consulted, and all the operations you've undergone?…

Good. What does all that say to you?… I agree. It's been a terrible journey of hope followed by disappointment, like searching for the holy grail or something, and you are right, modern medicine has not done a lot for you. But I just want to say that medicine is an imperfect thing. With all the things we see on television, it does sometimes leave both doctors and patients with a feeling that medicine should have all the answers. But the harsh reality is that it doesn't. I agree, no one has been able to cure you. And I think you're also saying that every time things got a little bit worse, your family practitioner referred you for another scan that never really got to the bottom of things. And every time you saw another specialist, he did another test or cut another piece out of your body and still your symptoms did not change much or it got worse. … I really am amazed at how much modern medicine has put you through for so little improvement in your pain.

The practitioner could capitalize on the rapport established through this genuine exposition of concern, and try a modified pros and cons strategy.

Practitioner: Turning again to the new, enhanced scan, I want you to try and think of some of the advantages of having the scan, and then I want you to try and tell me about some of the reasons why a scan might not be the best option right now.

Patient: Well, the most obvious thing is that the scan might find out what is causing my pain, and once we know, we may be able to cure it. On the other hand, it could be like all the others; a lot of trouble and radiation for little benefit to me. To tell you the honest truth, I'm sick of going back and forward to the hospital. I think they see me coming and say, *Oh no, here she comes again*, but I tell you, it's their fault. If they had taken me seriously in the first place, I wouldn't be like this now.

The patient is diverging from the pros and cons strategy and beginning to engage in a blaming exercise. This diverts energy away from the patient as the most important factor in shaping the future. Pinpointing fault is impossible and usually fruitless. The practitioner therefore avoids any discussion about blame. The practitioner might provide some generalized information and ask the patient to interpret.

Practitioner: I was reading in a medical journal the other day about people who have had numerous operations over the years without any improvement in their symptoms. They found that discovering a physical cause for the pain that could be put right almost never happened with such people. The people who did best were those who started finding their own solutions rather than continuing to look to medicine to cure them. What do you make of this research?

If this leads nowhere, try to reinforce the implicit message, while at the same time expressing concern and flexibility. Remember, if this patient leaves your office dissatisfied, she will find another practitioner who will send her for the scan and when her symptoms are not relieved, this new practitioner is likely to tire of her and she will move on, trapped in a perpetual cycle of hope and disappointment, and never seeing beyond the false grail of a biomedical quick fix.

Practitioner: OK, well, like you, I can see good and bad sides to the scan. Now I'm not saying that I won't refer you for the scan under any circumstances, and I want you to know that I will do my best to provide you with the finest ongoing medical care. But I want to see the thing in perspective and see you as a whole person, not just as a collection of symptoms. Sometimes, taking time out from the ongoing saga of tests and trying to answer the question, *How can I live with the problem a little better?* as opposed to finding an absolute cure can be a good thing. But let's both keep an open mind. Returning to your pain, I wonder if we could make a list of some of the things that are associated with it being a bit worse, and some of the things that you can do which seem to ease it a bit?

Here the practitioner may use a modified agenda-setting chart, where things which are, to a certain extent at least, under the patient's control (e.g., medications, communication with her partner, exercise, diet, distractions) are put in blank circles. Simply listing things that the patient could be in control of may be therapeutic in itself. The patient then selects one area to work on. Importance and confidence are then assessed in relation to this behavior, which could lead into using the useful scaling questions, brainstorming solutions, and setting attainable goals.

Practitioner: Why don't we leave it at that then for today? What you have told me today confirms in my mind how hard you are trying to cope with a bad situation. I like your idea of talking to your husband about your pain each day for about 5 or 10 min only, and then making sure that you have quality time together to talk and plan about other things which have nothing to do with your pain. Let me know how this has gone when we meet again in 2 weeks.

KEY POINTS

Empathy rather than resistance is the way through here. If you can understand, and show that you understand, the frustration and desperation at the root of the requests, you may be able to have a more collaborative conversation about the options.

Shifting focus from external magic bullets to acceptance and personal control.

REFERENCES

Butler, C.C., Pill, R., Stott, N.C.H., 1998. A qualitative study of patients' perceptions of doctors' advice to quit smoking: implications for opportunistic health promotion. British Medical Journal 316, 1878–1881.

Miller, W.R., Rollnick, S., 2012. Motivational Interviewing: Helping People Change, third ed. Guilford Press, New York.

Sesney, J.W., Kreher, N.E., Hickner, J.M., Webb, S., 1997. Smoking cessation interventions in rural family practices: an UPRNet study. Journal of Family Practice 44, 578–585.

Learning to practice this approach

10

CHAPTER OUTLINE

INTRODUCTION

This book focuses on helping people to consider making changes in their daily lives. One of the key messages has been that people change when it is *important* to them to do so and they feel *confident* about being able to achieve it. There are probably some parallel processes at work for practitioners learning to apply this approach to their work. If you have gotten as far as reading this chapter, you are probably interested in this way of working and wondering if it is important enough to you to apply it to your own practice. How confident you feel may depend on how different this approach is to the way you already work and how far you feel you have transferable skills.

HOW DO ADULTS LEARN TO ADAPT THEIR WORKING PRACTICES?

As a reader of this book, you are probably someone who absorbs information and ideas well through reading. How else do you learn well?

- Reading is accessible and flexible in terms of how much you do and when.
- Some people find it more helpful to have someone else explain ideas to them through lectures and talks. Making notes and having supporting material provided can reinforce this and help with retention of the information.
- "Sitting next to Nellie" is a traditional way of learning related to the apprenticeship model where we learn by observing others. Medical professionals will recall the old adage of "see one, do one, teach one," with observation being the first stage. This, of course, only works when there is a competent colleague to observe, and some practitioners are luckier than others in this respect.
- Use of audio–visual examples (on DVD, CD-ROM, etc.) can be an alternative to watching someone do it live and has the advantage that parts of the consultation can be watched again.
- Practicing (either in vivo or in a simulated situation) under the supervision of a more experienced colleague is one way in which most of us have honed our skills, especially in the early days of professional development. Such supervisors can help us with both positive and negative reinforcement.
- Reflective practice is an increasingly popular way to learn. Journals and face-to-face discussion sessions with peers can help us to observe more clearly what we are doing and to what effect. We deliver our own reinforcements through this process and then do more of the things that work or feel good and less of the things that do not. Reflective practice encourages a greater mindfulness in the way we work.
- New ways of working are often developed through experimentation, which clearly needs to be supported by reflective practice.

People all learn differently and usually respond well to the use of more than one method: for example, hearing a lecture, then seeing a demonstration, and then trying to do it with someone else's coaching. Ultimately, we learn to do by doing.

WHAT IMPEDES YOUR LEARNING OF THIS APPROACH?

Over a few years of teaching this approach, we have come across various obstacles to people's learning. Some people are reasonably satisfied with the way they are working at present, so there is just not enough motivation to try something different. When some of their patients do not take advice to change health behaviors, they attribute this to characteristics of the patients or their circumstances rather than to the style of the consultation. If you have been interested enough to read so far, this probably does not apply to you. You are wondering if you might be able to do something differently with better results.

Some people are just too busy to be able to "see the forest for the trees" in their jobs. They attend a lecture or workshop or read an article, are interested and engaged with the ideas, but then get overwhelmed with the volume of their workload. Even though a new style of working might ease their workload in the long term by enabling patients to take more responsibility for their own health and well-being, in the short term, it is quicker to conduct "business as usual" so the ideas get forgotten.

Increasingly, health practitioners are set targets to meet. For example, a smoking cessation service might be given targets of seeing X people in a year, getting X% of them to set a quit date, and X% of these to abstain from smoking for at least a month. Such practitioners feel under pressure and find it more difficult to maintain a patient-centered approach. They start thinking:

> We can't spend [waste?] time asking people how they feel about their smoking. We have to get them to quit and if they don't want to quit now, we need to stop working with them and find some more people who do want to quit.

Being in such a situation makes it very difficult for practitioners to embrace the spirit of this approach and to value the time they spend with patients who are still contemplating change.

Linked to this is what William Miller calls the *righting reflex*. This is the "powerful desire to set things right, to heal, to prevent harm, and to promote well being" (Rollnick et al., 2008). The righting reflex can seriously get in the way of "rolling with resistance" and can lead to a firm advice-giving stance. Even practitioners experienced in using this approach struggle to keep their righting reflex at bay! Where it is very strong, it can make it difficult to believe that an approach such as this is appropriate, and this gets in the way of learning how to do it.

The learning environment can hinder the process. A certain level of stress or arousal is useful in keeping the brain active and focused, but too much anxiety gets in the way of learning. Practicing new skills (or new ways of using old skills) is best done in a nonjudgmental and safe environment. Good coaches or mentors are supportive rather than critical and use a mix of positive and negative reinforcements.

Sometimes, health professionals say things to themselves or their colleagues that make learning less likely:

- *I'll learn this in a 1-day workshop.* It would be great if it were true. A workshop will certainly familiarize you with the ideas and set you on the path to learning the skills. Real proficiency with any skill comes over time, practicing in a range of different situations, being mindful all the time of what works well and learning from mistakes. The feedback you get from your patients' responses will be your best teacher if you pay attention to it. If you do not have access to a workshop that you can attend in person, you can learn through distance learning, practice, and peer support.

- *Role-play is artificial.* Yes of course it is! Some people do not like it for this reason. They feel that they *perform* less well in a role-play situation than they would in real life. This may be true, but it may not matter if it still teaches you something about what works well and what works badly. One of the most common comments we have had as trainers, running workshops, is, *I hate role-play but I must admit it was the most useful part of the course.* Playing the part of the patient is particularly instructive in developing a "feel" for resistance and readiness to change. It may sometimes be appropriate to use "real play" instead. In real play, rather than role-playing a patient and health professional, the participants use a real issue that one of them presents and work as colleagues addressing this issue using the techniques described in that section of the workshop.

- *This is nothing new, I do this every day.* If the basics feel familiar to you, it may be that you would enjoy exploring some of the more subtle aspects. There are lots of work to be done in refining this approach, improving the way we ask questions, developing more sophisticated reflections, and adapting all of this to patients from different cultural and ethnic groups presenting with different attitudes to their own behavior change. Trainers and educators have found it particularly stimulating explaining this approach to students and junior colleagues. They often ask perceptive questions, uncovering for us the aspects about which we all need to learn more.

- *Listening is easy; you just sit back and let them talk.* It is said that nature abhors a vacuum, and it is amazing what your head fills up with when you think you have opened your mind to listening to someone! Staying focused is a real skill needing constant vigilance. We have found that maintaining a curious manner helps. Some people find that their biggest temptation is to jump in with helpful suggestions; others that they want to interrupt to reassure patients and take the worry and uncertainty away. These are worthy aims but do obstruct the listening process.

- *I don't have the time for this, I have other more important things to do.* It is always helpful to have in mind the difference between *urgent* and *important*. Sometimes we all fail to make time for important work because we feel overwhelmed trying to keep up with urgent things, some of which are not really all that important.

At the very beginning of this book, we gave a few examples of patients who trigger frustration and feelings of inadequacy. You might like to do a quick count of how many patients like that you saw last week and use that as a marker to consider how important it is to you to make time to explore new ways of working. Once you decide it is important, it might be easier to make time.

It certainly can take longer to help people resolve their own problems compared with offering them a readymade solution. There is an old saying that if you give a man a fish, you feed him for a day; if you teach him to fish, you feed him for the rest of his life. This kind of work is more like teaching someone to fish or even helping them to discover that they had the skills to fish all along!

WHAT HELPS YOUR LEARNING OF THIS APPROACH?

People can grasp ideas by reading about them or being taught in a formal setting, but they develop their skills in the workplace. It has been found particularly helpful when a whole team or at least two or three people have embarked on a process of learning this approach. They can support each other, work together to resolve difficulties, and ensure the environment is conducive to learning. Occasional meetings with an external facilitator to refresh or update learning are sometimes possible in such a setting.

It is easier to learn something when you can link it with something you already know or can do. As you have been reading this book, you have probably been identifying things you already do well, and it is helpful to validate these as well as challenging yourself to try new things. You have probably also been relating the theory to patients currently or previously on your caseload, or even to your own experiences of personal behavior change. This is a great way to consolidate learning and will help you to retain it.

Internalizing the spirit of this approach helps considerably in becoming fluent with the techniques. Taking time to think about, and talk through with colleagues, the principles of personal choice and the role of the health professional can help, as can being vigilant about making some of the *dangerous assumptions* mentioned in Chapter 2. Practitioners attending workshops frequently say that discussion of these ideas is the thing that will make most difference to their practice.

Finally, an excellent way to clarify and consolidate new ideas is to explain them to someone else. Giving a presentation at a team meeting or writing an article for the practice newsletter can help you to marshal your thoughts and identify what you really have learned through your reading, workshop attendance, etc.

There has not been research specifically into how people learn this approach, but research into how people learn motivational interviewing (Miller and Mount, 2001) found that a 2-day workshop alone did not increase people's competence sufficiently, but when feedback on performance or coaching was added, they became proficient.

TEACHING YOURSELF THROUGH PRACTICE
SPIRIT AND TECHNIQUE

To become bogged down in matters of technique and strategy can lead one away from the more important spirit of these consultations about behavior change. The variety of techniques that could be used is almost endless, but as noted in Chapter 2, the spirit is more enduring. Some practitioners will want more structure to guide their work than others and are looking for some more tools for their toolbox.

The metaphor of a toolbox has its limitations. In truth, while the tasks we have identified are clearly defined, the strategies are not really like tools in a toolbox because one will always want to adapt and refine them to suit the individual.

PRACTICE

A 3- to 5-min consultation in an emergency room with an alcohol user will be different from a 20-min review of multiple behaviors with a patient who has chronic diabetes. This method covers a broad area. You need to ask yourself, *How does it fit into my context?* Some parts will be useful; others less so or even irrelevant. As an individual practitioner, trying things out with patients will do them no harm because of the emphasis placed on active, empathic listening in the method. You will soon learn what suits your patients, your context, and your consulting style.

CONSIDER A MENU

We have structured the method described in previous chapters around a set of tasks that follow a roughly sequential order in a consultation. One does not necessarily need to be restricted by this structure. One useful starting point is simply to construct a menu of strategies that you consider important for application in your everyday work. We have observed groups of colleagues readily reaching consensus about what tasks match their needs and what a provisional menu of strategies might look like. Some menus might have a stronger sequential order than others. The outcome is freedom for practitioners to choose a strategy at any given moment in the consultation.

YOUR PATIENT IS THE BEST TEACHER

Once your conversation begins, trying out a new approach can remind you of the experience of learning to drive a car. You focus so much on the little changes that it's difficult to see the way ahead. One of the most liberating experiences comes from the effect of asking a good open question; it gives you a little breathing space, so you can listen to the patient and even consider the way ahead. When this happens, you can take advantage of probably the most powerful way of learning, from the reaction of the patient. If the patient seems engaged, you are doing well. If you adopt a curious attitude to the body language and words used by the patient, you can use these cues to guide you and the patient to the next step or task. If the patient seems disengaged, try not to continue with the same tack but either shift focus or share your understanding with the patient about how they might be feeling. Perhaps they know what might be useful to discuss.

STOP! DO YOU KNOW WHAT YOU ARE DOING RIGHT NOW?

This is a useful general guideline. If you are working skillfully, you should be able to stop in the middle of a conversation and have a sense of what you are doing, why and how the patient is reacting to the structure you are providing and the strategy you have employed. This does not mean that the conversation should be full of flawless promises to change behavior. Indeed, you and the patient might be very confused about where to go next. But you should at least be aware that this is happening and have a sense of where to go next in the consultation. You do not need to have all the answers about behavior change, but you should at least be able to manage the consultation. If confused, you can sometimes be frank with the patient to remarkably good effect.

SKILLFUL PRACTITIONERS DO NOT ALWAYS PLAY BY THE RULES!

Practitioners might need to apply these strategies in a relatively mechanical way to begin with, much as one does when learning to drive. Things can feel clumsy and a bit forced. In these circumstances, it would be unwise to blame yourself, or the strategies, if all that is happening is that you are learning about your, and their, potential and limitations.

Practitioners who learn these strategies and practice them hard eventually stop slavishly following the recommendations and guidelines here. They get halfway through a strategy, leap on to another, return to where they left off, try something completely new, and so on. Observation soon reveals that this is creative adaptation of the highest caliber. Usually, however, they will say that they had some clumsy struggles to begin with. They will also report that the decision about what strategy to use next, often taken during a very brief pause in the conversation, requires more mental agility than the execution of the strategies themselves. The key is maintaining the spirit.

SKILLFUL PRACTITIONERS STICK TO SIMPLE THINGS

Shortly before retiring, a hospital physician colleague said, *Thirty years of experience has taught me to ask fewer questions, simpler questions, and to listen very carefully to the answers.* This practitioner knew what simple open questions to use at the right time. Perhaps even more important, she apparently knew what to leave out, what was not essential to the fruitful conduct of the consultation. Another colleague likened this process to the art of good cooking. His observation of a famous Chinese chef on television led him to observe, *It all looks so easy; this cook just throws a few simple ingredients together. But it is deceptive. He knows what to leave out, and that must have taken a lot of practice.*

SPLIT YOURSELF IN HALF

It is obviously worthwhile to have your attention focused firmly on the patient. This is the art of active, empathic listening. You also need to have some of your attention focused on what is happening between the two of you, how the patient is reacting, and where you are at the level of strategy. This challenge is obviously not unique to talk about behavior change but is an essential part of skillful helping and consulting of all kinds. You move along two trajectories at the same time.

WHAT TO EXPECT FROM A TRAINING WORKSHOP

A training workshop alone is unlikely to be all you need, but for many people, it is a good start. You might expect any of the following: a new slant on an old problem of "patient noncompliance," inspiration to try something different, clarification of ideas about which you have already read, coaching in skills, or discussion with peers interested in the same ideas.

Below is a list of objectives that might have been set by the workshop facilitator. By the end of the workshop or educational program, they might be planning that you will be able to

- describe a model for understanding changing lifestyle behaviors
- raise the issue of lifestyle change with a patient in a way that does not elicit resistance
- use an agenda-setting strategy to help patients decide what changes they might talk about
- use the model and associated visual aids to assess a patient's feelings about change (readiness, importance, and confidence)
- assist a patient in exploring the importance of a particular behavior change and the confidence to achieve it
- use a range of active listening skills to enable a patient to clarify his or her own feelings about lifestyle change
- conduct a consultation in such a way as to leave the responsibility for change, and the right to decide whether or not to change, clearly with the patient
- give accurate and appropriate information about lifestyle and health in a neutral way and enable patients to interpret the implications for their own situation
- describe how you handle your own frustrations when working with patients who do not, at present, want to change and how you avoid attempting to impose your own timetable for change on the patient
- describe an overview of the method's tasks and strategies
- use a menu of strategies for guiding the consultation

A good workshop will use a variety of training methods and will include opportunities for practice. Retention of learning is related to practice, and we learn best, even in formal situations, when we can actively participate.

A good workshop facilitator will make the training relevant to participants' work contexts and give appropriate demonstrations and practice opportunities. It is not always easy to tell from brochures or websites how good training will be, and there is no system at present for accrediting trainers in this area. Word of mouth is the way many people choose a course.

There is no accreditation or licensing process for practitioners in this approach (although a workshop may be taught as part of a bigger program that carries accreditation). You can learn it in whatever way you choose and practice it in whichever way you find works best. Research will continue to guide you in this.

OTHER STRUCTURED LEARNING OPPORTUNITIES

Finally, here are a few innovations in practice that we have observed among practitioners in different settings, all geared toward improving the outcome of conversations about behavior change:

- *Peer support meetings.* Practitioners can present interesting cases in turn, with an emphasis on experiences of success to begin with. Some groups even consider presenting new strategies and trying these out in role-play form. Others have formed a study group, where they discuss new ideas or articles about their kind of service, or even view videotapes of good practice.
- *Individual or group supervision.* An experienced practitioner-trainer meets regularly with team members to consider their progress, even using audiotapes of consultations as the platform for learning.
- *Team meetings.* There is huge potential in meetings of the entire team to consider anything from improvements to the service as a whole to how best to enhance consultation practice. These two options are not disconnected because between them sit a range of procedures and practices that have direct bearing on behavior change.
- *Use of multimedia.* A DVD and CD learning pack has been developed by the authors of this book and its previous editions. This provides short demonstrations accompanied by worksheets to complete while watching (Mason and Butler, 2010). This is appropriate for private study or teaching purposes.

One team we worked with redesigned their assessment so that both question content and the procedure itself were more in line with promoting behavior change. Another team examined the sequence of procedures that patients went through and decided that behavior change would be more likely to occur if patients had choice about the order of activities they went through.

One of the most innovative changes we have observed arose from a decision to conduct a simple survey of patients with diabetes to ascertain their views about the service. It emerged that they found it difficult to get to the clinic and tiring to be "lectured" about lifestyle change. This ultimately led to the relocation of the clinic into the community and to staff becoming much more flexible in the way they approached the topic of behavior change.

REFERENCES

Mason, P., Butler, C., 2010. Ready, Willing and Able; Helping Patients to Consider Behaviour Change. Pip Mason Consultancy Ltd., Birmingham UK. www.pipmason.com.

Miller, W.R., Mount, K.A., 2001. A small study of training in motivational interviewing: does one workshop change clinician and client behavior? Behavioral and Cognitive Psychotherapy 29, 457–471.

Rollnick, S., Miller, W.R., Butler, C.C., 2008. Motivational Interviewing in Health Care: Helping Patients Change Behavior. Guilford Press, New York.

Calls from the consulting room

11

CHAPTER OUTLINE

LISTENING A LITTLE, HELPING A LOT

This book has described quite a few things you can do with patients when talking about behavior change, all based on the idea that your skillfulness can make a big difference to outcome. The most fundamental perhaps is listening. Here is a slightly unusual true story from a hospital ward where the behavior change involved agreeing to undergo surgery. A little listening transformed a seemingly desperate situation:

She completely refuses to have surgery. The patient refused to agree to cardiac surgery despite a warning that she could die soon after returning home if she did not. Two surgeons and a nurse tried to persuade her. Their approach was based on rational persuasion; two of them tried a soft and kind approach to information-giving, while the third, perhaps feeling a little desperate, tried to induce fear by pointing out how grim the prognosis was if she did not agree.

Then a nurse decided to wait until the patient had had an afternoon nap to "have a quiet word." She came alongside the patient and did not try to persuade her. The episode of listening took 5–7 min. It turned out that the patient wanted to be discharged because she wanted to be with her partner. The nurse offered to call her partner and ask him to come in and talk things through. His increased presence and support over the following 24 h led to a joint decision to undergo surgery.

CAN LISTENING DO HARM?

The successful resolution to the surgery example discussed above started with a simple question: *How are you feeling*? Listening led to the solution. Yet calls do come from the consulting room that are not so straightforward. One of the most common is a concern that listening can place both the practitioner and patient in a difficult position. Here is an example.

The patient

He was 35 years old, had type I diabetes and worked as a barman, smoking and drinking, and leading a "work hard, play hard" kind of existence. He did worry about his control of his diabetes, particularly when he would have what he called a *hypo*, get irritable, and throw people out of the bar. His daily routine was seldom predictable, and he often went out to parties after work.

The setting

Like many patients with long-term conditions, this man went to his routine outpatient consultation with an air of resignation. He expected what he called, *the usual lecture about my bad behavior.*

The consultation

The nurse asked him how he was getting on, making a genuine attempt to listen, because she had 25 min set aside for him; she had met him once before. He started responding to her genuine interest in his everyday life. He said the structure of his life was all messed up and his diabetes often got neglected. *Hypos* caused trouble. His smoking was something he clung to; it made him feel in control and helped in all kinds of moods. The nicest thing was that the first puff was a time to take a break from it all, a moment to rest. They were 8 min into the consultation when she offered a listening statement, a summary of her understanding of what he was saying.

Nurse: In all these busy times, it's like you're in the fast lane and you find it hard to slow down.
Patient: Exactly right. I can't and it's a darned mess.
Nurse: And your smoking, you say it's just part of this life.
Patient: Completely. I can't imagine doing without it.
Nurse: It's like your best friend.
Patient: [Puts his head in both hands, looks up] This is a ridiculous mess. [Bursts into sobbing and puts his head down again]

What's going on here? Has this high-quality listening been harmful? What should she do now? This real case example was discussed with a multidisciplinary team, and their conclusions were as follows:

- They often came across people like this, felt very concerned about them, and usually did not know how to deal with them. One tendency was for them to pass this kind of case from one professional to another, in the hope that someone else might do better than they could.
- Some staff felt that it was not part of their role to do this kind of counseling, while the majority felt that it was an inevitable part of their work. One nurse put it this way: *You never know which patient is teetering on the edge of despair until it's too late. You can't avoid it.*
- Listening is part of quality health care. Practitioners should not shy away from this.
- The experience of being listened to could be the turning point for many patients. If handled well, they will feel cared for and appreciative.
- A distressed patient does not necessarily need to have a problem solved. The nurse need not feel that anything needs to be fixed. Her genuineness is key.
- Among the potentially useful possibilities in a case like this were to comfort him and then summarize the situation, to offer affirmation in a genuine manner, to see if he wanted to talk about any changes to his lifestyle, and to offer support and a commitment to seeing him again.

The enormous potential value of listening in a case like this, and so many others, cannot be underestimated. It is only with considerable insensitivity in response to an upset patient that harm can be done. The most important thing that patients need in this kind of situation is a sense of being contained and supported. They do not necessarily want practical advice, and it's usually quite straightforward to round up an episode of listening by summarizing what has been said, offering a few supportive observations and asking permission to change direction.

Most practitioners know the experience of listening to a patient and wondering where it will end. When patients feel listened to, they can sometimes experience a hunger for more, leaving you concerned about time and how to bring matters to a constructive close. The few simple guidelines noted above are usually sufficient to deal with most situations.

YOUR EMOTIONS

Talking about behavior change is no neutral matter, where one can sit in a comfortable and detached bubble and just get on with the job. Emotions can run high. Frustration is common because you cannot make people change, yet you often feel strong that if only the patient would change, their health would improve.

Those shoes she wears are a big problem; yet she refuses to change them, even though she knows that surgery might be necessary if she does not. (Podiatrist)

When I ask them about using condoms I get this shrug, even though we both know that HIV/AIDS is a problem around here. (Nurse, South Africa)

If frustration is the outcome, other emotions often provide the starting point: concern for the patient's well-being, optimism about making a difference, or sometimes even desperation about helping someone to avoid trouble looming in the future. Patients, for their part, often resist openly or "close down" in response to strong urging from the practitioner. They have their own views about their lives and can be left feeling guilty, threatened, or even angry about your good intentions. This is because they probably sometimes feel that your best efforts threaten their autonomy to make decisions for themselves. Yet you cannot deny your feelings! Is there anything you can do that is constructive about this dilemma?

TAKE A STEP BACK

- How are you feeling, before, during, and after the consultation? Just knowing this can help. It settles you down. Self-awareness of this kind is an indication of professional and personal maturity. If you are in the middle of a consultation, it's often also the signal to change tack, to try something different.
- Are you falling into the trap of trying too hard to persuade the patient to change or of overloading them with information?
- Are you falling into the trap of just following the patient and getting nowhere? Are you losing control of the direction of the consultation?
- Remember, if you feel things are not going well, the chances are good that the patient will share that feeling.

ADJUST YOUR APPROACH

- Summarize what is been covered thus far. This is a good prelude to changing direction. See if you can capture how the patient is feeling and what he or she has said thus far about behavior change. Use *you* rather than *I* when doing this. Most patients will appreciate an effort to summarize in this way and would not mind you changing direction.
- Consider being open with the patient about what will be most helpful. Does the patient want you to provide advice, or does he or she just want to talk it through; in other words, have some space to consider the *why* and *how* of change (as outlined in this book)? The effect of this brief conversation will be to reinforce patients' sense of autonomy over decisions in their lives.
- Consider the menu of strategies outlined in this book. Their purpose is to allow you to stand back in a relatively more neutral position, while you guide the patient through the process of considering the *why* and *how* of change.

TALK WITH COLLEAGUES

Serious professional work of any kind requires a proper context for education, supervision, and professional development. The consultation about behavior change deserves the same attention to quality as any other aspect of treatment. At the heart of this process is talking with colleagues and reflecting about how to improve your own well-being and that of your patients.

> Over time, because we talked openly about our consultations and patient education activities, I noticed something: there was a lot less frustrating talk around the place about *should*, *must*, and *ought to* when it came to patient behavior change. Our attitude had begun to change, and we were focused more on our skills than what patients should or should not do. (Doctor, cardiac rehabilitation unit)

In busy health-care settings, there is no shortage of things that cause strain for practitioners. Getting through a busy clinic can be tiring enough without the sometimes arduous matter of keeping records, attending meetings, following protocols, and so on. These forces affect morale and well-being, and they affect one's conduct in the conversation about behavior change. Usually, this takes the form of slipping into a default style that involves persuading and "educating" patients about the need to change. One of the constructive effects of using the strategies outlined in this book is that, in time, and with skill, you do not have to fall into a morale-sapping default routine. Each patient is unique. Each has the solution to behavior change within them. You do not have to take responsibility for solving the problem. You elicit this from them in a supportive atmosphere. This is better for your morale as well. You might get to feel less frustrated; you will notice outcomes improving for your patients.

SOME PATIENTS LIKE TO BE TOLD WHAT TO DO

All practitioners can tell stories about patients who are passive and expectant of expert opinion. Indeed, in many cultures, this kind of passivity is required of the person consulting a healer, witch doctor, or health practitioner. Surely the more negotiation-based method described here is inappropriate for some people, who perhaps might not want to take responsibility for sharing decision-making. Unfortunately, we have not found a brief method for assessing at the outset of a discussion whether or not a patient likes to be told what to do when it comes to behavior change. If we had, we would be in a much better position to understand how many people feel this way, in what circumstances and how best to respond to them.

Care should be taken not to polarize the difference between advice-giving and a more negotiation-based approach to behavior change. This issue was discussed in Chapter 2. We have all given advice and told people what they should do without undermining their autonomy. Often this depends on how you say things. Similarly, we have also felt free to say what we think patients should do while using a more negotiation-based framework. The key is to make sure that we emphasize their freedom to make a decision for themselves. In truth, if you have sufficiently good rapport with patients, you can usually offer your opinion without any harm being done. The concern about advice-giving is that it should not be the default style for behavior change consultations because too many patients do not respond well. If you feel that a particular patient wants to be told what to do, try it and be wary of triggering resistance. If you are not sure, ask the patient.

SOME PATIENTS WILL NEVER CHANGE

Why should I be so optimistic about change? Some of my patients will never be able to. (Dietitian, aged 42)

This kind of question echoes through our minds in every clinic, and the answer, we believe, is in the rejection of dogmatism. The problem is this: we are often quick to pass judgment and we are often wrong. For example, a team of three counselors once made a rating of each of 142 male heavy drinkers at the receiving end of a hospital-based health promotion effort, i.e., 0 = very unlikely to change; 5 = very likely to change. Follow-up at 6 months revealed no relationship between their judgments and outcome. Some of the "hopeless cases" did very well.

Yet we all know cases where our intuitions are borne out by seeing the same person, time after time, never changing. For example, a 55-year-old obese woman has been suffering, like her father before her, with the complications of diabetes. She routinely attends the clinic, submits herself to all the measurements, yet develops a blank look whenever one talks about dietary change. She struggles with a stressful and economically deprived lifestyle and, like her father before her, does not appear to believe that it is possible or worthwhile to slow the progress of the disease. The family value system is like a brick wall, and one shudders at the thought of what medical crisis might befall her.

It is one thing to feel resigned about a particular patient, but care should be taken in generalizing too much about peoples' chances, lest we develop hardened or cynical attitudes that are not in the interests of good practice. The approach described in this book is not a panacea imbued with healing powers to resolve problems like those described in the example above. It is, however, an approach that calls for flexibility and the avoidance of dogmatism.

THEY KNOW ALL THE FACTS BUT THEY NEVER LISTEN, THEY NEVER CHANGE

This is probably the most frequently vented frustration in the treatment of chronic diseases such as asthma, heart disease, and diabetes. Patients are not short of information — in fact, they often hear the same story about "looking after yourself" in every clinic — yet they make very little progress in altering lifestyle habits.

There is obviously no single explanation or single answer to this problem. We have been very impressed by the way in which practitioners sometimes take a deep breath and decide to have an open discussion about the matter. The strategies in this book are merely aids to this activity (e.g., agenda setting, exploring importance). Perhaps the most surprising issue uncovered by these practitioners is that the patient is struggling not with behavior change but with the meaning of the chronic disease itself. The case of Marco is a good example of this.

Marco suffers from what the doctors and nurses call *asthma*. He has been coming to the clinic for some years and regularly hears talk about behavior change. For example, *Remember not only to take your inhaler, but also the other medicine* [a prophylactic steroid]. Marco seldom takes this advice. The practitioners feel frustrated about his poor compliance and apparent irrationality.

Many patients like Marco have concerns about what they see as the dangers in taking a particular medicine like a steroid. This is not a particularly deep underlying issue, and one is left wondering whether the patient's concerns about taking medicine are dealt with through information exchange in a sufficiently thorough manner at the point of diagnosis. More serious, however, is the fact that Marco does not agree that he has asthma in the first place. He calls it his *bad chest*. Lack of agreement about the meaning and implications of a diagnosis could account for quite a lot of poor compliance, something which came to light in a recent study of patients with asthma (Adams et al., 1997). Time spent talking with Marco about exactly what the diagnosis means and how this fits into his everyday life might have prevented so much time and effort being wasted in repeated exhortations to take his medication as prescribed. The focus by the clinic staff on behavior change (taking medication) was clearly premature in Marco's case. Practitioners were prematurely talking about behavior change when Marco did not see the "disease" in the same way as them.

Along similar lines, another man had been diagnosed with type I diabetes at the age of 11 years. Until very recently, this 55-year-old man had been ignoring his disease, trying to live life despite it, as he put it, *messing around with my insulin levels*. On his own admission, he behaved like an irritable and obnoxious person when he went to his routine clinic. He hated the way *they* were obsessed by insulin levels. Then recently, a nurse and doctor decided that his physical condition was so serious that they had to take a different approach, give him more time, and allow him to talk about whatever he wanted. They said that he had been in a state of denial for over 40 years, not able to see the connection between his condition and his health problems. He said that they had now given him help, not lectures, and that they had taken him into the real world where he felt much more in control of what he wanted from life.

The lesson seems clear enough; if patients repeatedly fail to listen and to change, it might be worthwhile listening to them, without prejudice, to give them a chance to say what truly underlies their apparent disengagement from the agenda of the practitioner.

A LITTLE BIT OF KNOWLEDGE CAN BE DANGEROUS

I attended a workshop and you encouraged me to examine why my patients are unsure about change. I did this, unpacked a lot of personal issues, and then I got stuck and did not know how to end the brief consultation effectively. Don't you think that's dangerous? (Community nurse, aged 27)

At least three issues emerge from this comment, each worthy of being taken seriously. These are, first, that we might endanger patients by opening a "can of worms" that we cannot deal with; second, that practitioners might be harmed by feeling out of their depth; and third, that a one-off training experience can leave practitioners feeling inadequately supported.

First, one can imagine a scenario in which concern about harming patients is legitimate. A practitioner with poor communication skills uses a behavior change strategy like a dose of intervention with a poor sense of timing and judgment and leaves the patient feeling upset. We have taken care to emphasize the spirit of this method (Chapter 2), which is based on listening carefully and working with the readiness to change of the patient. As such, used with a modicum of skill, it can do patients no harm. The nurse described above is not likely to do any harm because he or she is asking questions of his or her own consulting behavior and watching the reaction of the patients. The chances are that the nurse's judgment will improve with time, experience, and support.

The second issue, practitioners feeling out of their depth, is a serious challenge that faces trainers and supervisors. Use of this approach can and does leave practitioners feeling out of their depth at times. One nurse said that it took about a year before he or she felt comfortable with an adjustment to his or her consulting style and felt at home with a more flexible approach to behavior change. During this period, he or she struggled. Fortunately, someone had the opportunity to talk to him or her about his or her experiences, which were as much positive as negative. The main difficulty was how to handle a situation in which both parties realized that there was no way out of an impasse; it simply was not the right time to consider change. This colleague's resolution of this problem involved feeling free to summarize the situation for the patient and to offer reassurance that change takes time, that it is better to think things over before rushing into a decision. The battle was with his or her own sense of impotence to solve patients' problems for them. Feeling out of one's depth is probably a call for more supervision and training, not for a return to simple advice-giving.

The third problem, providing inadequate, one-off training, is a pervasive one, particularly in a relatively new field which has not been integrated into the basic training of practitioners in a widespread manner. However, the solution is probably not to stop conducting one-off training workshops but to run them in such a way that practitioners' concerns about skill levels are responded to with openness, reassurance, and some level-headed guidance about the sometimes tricky road ahead. If clinicians consider a workshop the best way for them to learn, as discussed in Chapter 10, they will be able to develop their practice despite the limitations of one-off training. The impetus for writing this book came from a desire to prompt curriculum designers to place the subjects of behavior change and information exchange close to the top of the list in the basic training of practitioners. Until that happens, the concerns of the nurse quoted above will be legitimate.

WHY SO MUCH TALK ABOUT BEHAVIOR? WHAT ABOUT FEELINGS?

The focus on behavior in this book might appear to have a narrow and somewhat arbitrary quality. How can one separate behavior from attitudes and feelings? Why develop strategies specifically for dealing with behavior in the absence of accompanying guidelines for dealing with these other domains? One answer to this is that one has to make a start somewhere. Practitioners spend a lot of time on the specific topic of behavior change, and we believe that the quality of this activity could be much improved. However, to view the tasks and strategies in this book as narrowly focused on behavior would be to misunderstand their function. We have described a number of concepts, principles, and strategies that help a practitioner to explore and acknowledge the way a patient is feeling and thinking. The patient-centered method is a critical foundation for ensuring that one does not stray into an oversimplified discussion of health behavior, removed from the personal context in which it occurs. Other concepts and strategies serve the same function; the observation of resistance, for example, is often a signal that the patient has other priorities. Asking a patient about the importance of change sometimes leads directly to the exploration of a more fundamental personal matter. The agenda-setting task was deliberately designed to encourage the patient to talk about other concerns beyond behavior change.

HOW DO HABITS AND ADDICTIONS FIT IN?

A long-term heavy user of diazepam will probably find it more difficult to change behavior than a young heavy drinker who is not dependent on alcohol. One of the differences between these two cases is in the degree of physical dependence on the substance. Remove the substance, and the diazepam user will experience withdrawal symptoms. Some people report severe symptoms that cripple their attempts to change and leave them feeling demoralized and trapped. Others, also apparently with a severe addiction, appear to find the transition from use to abstinence more straightforward. In the literature, debate about the meaning and ramifications of addiction has been smoldering for many years, particularly in the alcohol field (see Heather and Robertson, 1989). This is not merely an academic debate but one that has serious practical consequences.

Clearly, another inescapable difference between the long-term diazepam user and the young heavy drinker is in their degree of attachment to the substance, independent of any physical components of addiction. Here, we begin to move out of the realms of substance use. Do something for long enough, anything, and it can become a habit that is difficult to break. Sometimes the habit pervades many aspects of the person's daily life (e.g., gambling, drinking coffee, eating chocolate), and sometimes it is more circumscribed (e.g., brushing teeth). Obviously, the consequences vary across individuals and behaviors. As negative consequences emerge, if they do, the person can become embroiled in conflict about whether or not to change.

In general, addiction to substances can be viewed too narrowly as a matter of physical dependence, without sufficient emphasis being placed on habit strength and the patient's beliefs and moods. One of the consequences of this view, it could be argued, has been the emergence of specialists trained to help people through withdrawal and readjustment. This can be a double-edged sword. While intensive help is clearly extremely valuable for some people, particularly for those without active support in the community, it can reinforce the idea that a practitioner in a general health-care setting is in no position to deal with such matters. We question this assumption. There will never be enough specialists to deal with the number of addictive problems that appear in primary and other general health-care settings, something which policymakers have begun to take note of. Substance users, for their part, might not necessarily want the perceived stigma and inconvenience of specialist referral. Most important, however, is our belief that practitioners can make a great deal of progress within the limited time available to them. We have found it possible to use the approach in this book with patients suffering from severe addiction problems.

Most of these patients actually change their behavior quite naturally, without help from anyone. The method described in this book can be used as a starting point with any kind of problem, be it someone seriously dependent on benzodiazepines, a long-term heavy smoker, a severe problem drinker, or someone suffering from obesity. Whether this relatively brief input is sufficient is another matter, something for the patient and practitioner to decide. Establishing rapport, often in the face of considerable guilt and remorse, can be a powerful first step. Helping a patient express how he or she really feels about the issue (i.e., by assessing importance and confidence) can sometimes precipitate spontaneous change. For their part, practitioners need to hang on to the most important observation to emerge from the stages of change model: that action is not the only measure of success in a consultation. In fact, for the majority, this is inappropriate because they are not ready for this, let alone for accepting the idea of specialist referral. Helping someone think about change is a critical process, well within the capability of the general health-care practitioner. Addictive problems should not be mystified as being too complex. Whatever the degree of physical dependence, the challenges for the practitioner remain the same: establish rapport and have a constructive discussion about change.

CAN I USE THIS IN THE GROUPS THAT I RUN?

Some practitioners are already running groups in health-care settings that focus on behavior change. They wonder whether these groups could be based on the approach described in this book. Supporting evidence is lacking and our experience of this has been limited but sufficient to realize that this is a field rich in promise.

To run a group which focuses on a particular problem or behavior (e.g., diabetes, panic, alcohol) offers rich potential for promoting behavior change, as well as some serious traps that undermine autonomy and decision-making. The opportunities for observing the success of others and gaining their support are well-known and powerful forces in the self-help process. One temptation is to try to divide people up strictly into groups depending on their readiness to change. This can be useful, and there are services offering groups for precontemplators, contemplators, and so on. The problem here, not surprisingly, is that people jump in and out of stages quite easily. Each participant will be vulnerable at times to experiencing resistance when the group is moving further ahead than he or she feels ready for. We offer here a few thoughts on how to run groups in this style.

- Our approach to information exchange is usefully incorporated into a group because it encourages participants to respond personally to information presented in a neutral and nonthreatening way.
- Rolling with resistance, accompanied by a reflective listening style, is an excellent way to diffuse tension and discontent in a group. Once someone knows their antagonistic position has been heard and acknowledged, they are more likely to quieten down about it and, perhaps, feel free to move on.
- Monitor the style in which the group is run so that members' autonomy is supported, not threatened.
- Group assessments of readiness (on a continuum) can generate useful discussion. Participants could also use the importance and confidence dimensions in the same way. It can be fun to use these physically. Participants are asked to line-up in a continuum across the room on the particular dimension; for example, one

end of the room represents the highest importance of quitting smoking and the opposite end represents the lowest importance. Then, having lined-up in the room, people are asked to explain *Why so high?* They tell each other why they have chosen to be where they are rather than closer to the lower importance end of the room. They can also discuss, from this physical standpoint, what it would take to move them higher. This can get a little unruly but stimulates thought and raises energy.

- Exploration of ambivalence in a group can be tricky as the group can divide into two entrenched camps. An alternative to this is to have two chairs in the middle of the room, one representing the pros of a behavior and the other the cons. For example, a weight management group might have one chair representing reasons for incorporating regular exercise into a weight loss program and the other representing reasons not to bother with exercise. Participants are invited to sit in whichever chair they wish to support for a couple of minutes and debate with someone in the other. When someone else wants to join in, they tap the shoulder of the person they want to replace. It is acceptable, in fact desirable, for people to move from one seat to the other, giving them a chance to express both sides of their own ambivalence. If group leaders join in, they should take a turn in each seat to show that they appreciate both viewpoints.

- As with one-to-one work, the spirit and assumptions are crucial. Where the group leader truly trusts the participants to be able to make good decisions and find their own solutions to problems, the group takes on a different character. The group leader becomes a facilitator rather than an advisor, and the participants gain confidence by discovering their own resources and potential.

REFERENCES

Adams, S., Pill, R., Jones, A., 1997. Medication, chronic illness and identity; the perspective of people with asthma. Social Science and Medicine 45, 189–201.

Heather, N., Robertson, I., 1989. Problem Drinking, second ed. Oxford University Press, Oxford.

Example of a consultation

12

CHAPTER OUTLINE

Providing a case example carries risks, none more so than the idea that there is one ideal way of proceeding. The aim here is to provide a rough-and-ready illustration of how a consultation can unfold knowing that, just as in a musical rendition, mistakes are instructive and individual variation in emphasis is to be expected.

To approach authenticity, neither party was given a script for this consultation nor was there a rehearsal. Pip Mason took the role of a cardiac rehabilitation nurse, and the patient, an actor, was simply asked to imagine that he had suffered from a heart attack.

This transcript is taken from a training DVD (Gilligan and Mason, 2006). Commentary has been added, and you can watch the video clip via the website (http://evolve.elsevier.com/Mason/healthbehavior/). Whichever medium you start with, transcript or video, the commentary in this chapter should help to provide links between earlier chapters and clinical reality.

As you watch, you might want to ask yourself what the nurse's options were at each point and what would have been the likely outcome of doing something different. The foundation of skillfulness lies in the knowledge that each utterance of yours will affect what the patient says next. See what you think.

Nurse	OK Mr. Jenkins, what this appointment is about is to help you in any way that we can to think about how you are going to go on now you've had the heart attack and got over it, and any changes you want to make to stop it happening again. How are you feeling at the moment?	*Introduces agenda.* *Open question to establish rapport.*
David	Yes, I feel, you know, still a bit shaken by the whole thing, you know what I mean.	

Nurse	Frightening.	*Nurse is "logging" his first response carefully, paying attention to the words he uses and to the way he is feeling.*
David	Well it has come out of the blue a bit hasn't it? I didn't think people my age had heart attacks, you know what I mean.	
Nurse	No.	
David	Anyway, yes I am all right.	
Nurse	OK, so you are feeling OK in yourself, it's just kind of being in trepidation about the whole thing.	*Reflection (see p. 39) acknowledging feelings. She tries to capture his words and feelings in one utterance. The shorter the better. He used the word "shaken" and she used "trepidation."*
David	As I say, it's a bit, came as a bit of a shock to me.	*Elaborates as rapport builds.*
Nurse	What do you know about the risk factors for heart disease, about what might have contributed to you having the attack? How much do you know and how much of it has been explained already?	*Exchanging information as a precursor to setting the agenda. This is the first part of the "elicit—provide—elicit" strategy.*
David	Well I know it's like stuff about, you know, with my Dad. Dad had a heart attack. He died quite young.	*Begins to share what he already knows.*
Nurse	Right.	
David	So, that's something to do with it, isn't it?	
Nurse	Yes, it can run in families like that, yes.	
David	And umm, I've heard like, kind of stuff about me smoking and they are going to tell me to stop smoking. And, you know, all that sort of stuff I understand all that.	
Nurse	Yes, smoking is one of the things. What other things do you know of?	*Still exchanging information. Note that the patient has most of the information about risk factors already. The nurse merely provides supportive information as necessary.*

David	And drink, I think drink's part of it. Alcohol. I like a drink. I go for a drink usually every day after work, so, just sort of de-stress you know what I mean? Probably food as well isn't it? I like a burger. Which is probably the wrong thing to say isn't it?	*The patient provides the information, not the nurse. Defensiveness starting to creep in as he anticipates the way the consultation might go.*
Nurse	Well, basically it's best to be honest about how it is at the moment and try to think what you want to do, if you want to do anything different.	*Emphasizes his freedom of choice, even using the word "if."*
David	Yes, I suppose.	
Nurse	I mean, it sounds like you have got a bit of an idea of what it's all about. Some of the risk factors you can't do anything about. If it runs in your family, we can't do anything about that. It maybe just means that you might want to be extra careful in some of the sorts of things that you can control. There are some things that are controllable and some things aren't.	*Still exchanging information.*
David	Yes right, I can't change that then. You know, if my Dad has died of a heart attack.	
Nurse	No, you will always carry that extra propensity to it.	*Uses reflection rather than immediately jumping in to change he could make. This gives him the chance to take the discussion where he wants it to go.*
David	Right.	
Nurse	But it doesn't mean that it's inevitable that you will keep having heart attacks at all.	*Still exchanging information but now has moved the focus away from the behavior change agenda to reassurance as David is clearly very scared.*
David	OK.	
Nurse	No, I don't want you to go away with that idea that it's inevitable. And if your Dad died young, it doesn't mean you're going to die young. You haven't died of this one have you?	
David	No, I haven't no, but it shook me up somewhat.	
Nurse	Yes.	
David	You know what I mean; I don't want it to happen again.	

Nurse	Yes, a bit of a wake-up call.	*Reflection, subtly emphasizing, by using the expression "wake-up call," the fact that the fear might motivate him to think about how he is living at present.*
David	Terrifying yes, to think someone my age can have a heart attack, it's like — wake up one morning, that's it, you are going to have a heart attack. Flipping heck!	*If the nurse understates the feeling (a "bit" of a wake-up call), patients often amplify it ("Terrifying yes"). Usually best to understate rather than overstate.*
Nurse	Yes. Any other factors in your life that you think might contribute? Sometimes a lot of stress... I don't know what you do for a job, or other kinds of stresses?	*Guides the conversation back to agenda setting, perhaps prematurely.*
David	I have got stress coming out of my ears to be honest with you.	
Nurse	Tell me about that.	*Listening and following, moving toward exchanging information about stress.*
David	Well, I have got my own business haven't I, and it's just you know, running around, on the phone, on the computer. Doing about 10 people's jobs all at one time, you know. I am all over the area. I don't just stay in one place. I am driving around; I am making sure that the jobs are getting done. And I am taking phone calls from suppliers and you know what suppliers are like. I've a building company, you know what suppliers are like, they're a nightmare.	
Nurse	Yes.	*When following, the less said the better.*
David	You know what I mean. Just can't, they promise things and it doesn't turn up and then you have to get on the phone to them. And then it delays you on a job. And that delays you on the next job, and you've got people working for you lined up. It's just that, I'm getting stressed thinking about it.	

Nurse	It must have been really hard for you to suddenly be taken ill then.	*Expressing empathy not just with the stress of the job but also on the impact of his illness in the context of work.*
David	It's been a nightmare. You know, I've been off the last few weeks and I get back to, because there's no one covering for me if I am not there. Nothing happens is it. Mobile phone messages with the inbox's full, computer inbox's full. Just, yes, you know how it is.	*Elaborates as rapport continues to build.*
Nurse	So, in a sense when you're working for yourself, it's actually really important to keep in good health.	*Reframes his tale of woe about what happens when he is off work. It is reflected as change talk around the importance of keeping well.*
David	Well yes, people relying on me as well. You know what I mean. When I am not there, nothing happening. People sit around and, I don't know if we get paid or not. I got jobs lined up. Got knocked back and knocked back. And when it gets to summer, it's the busiest time; it gets to the winter and if I got jobs delayed. It's just, not good is it. So, yes I guess I have got to look after myself.	*Expresses the importance, as a businessman, of keeping well (goal established).*
Nurse	To keep your job, keep the business going.	*Reflection of importance in terms of his priorities, i.e., work.*
David	That's it, yes.	*The above reflection saved time because it summed up the patient's view of the problem. When he affirmed this, the nurse felt able to shift focus.*
Nurse	Let's have a look at some of the things that umm, that are possibly areas that you might want to do something about. Things that would help to prevent heart attacks. I will just kind of jot them down. The one we just talked about is work stress.	*Begins to use agenda-setting chart (see Appendices, p. 219).*
David	Yes.	
Nurse	Do you have any other sorts of stress that we need to be thinking about, that are going on for you?	

David	Not really. I have got kids and that, got a quite young family, you know. Demanding stuff all the time. Running around and if one of them's not well and that, you know. It stresses me out thinking that I'm, you know if I am going to be ill and they are only little. That gets me worried.	*Returns to talking about being scared. The practitioner's challenge at this point is to stay congruent with the fear and try and focus it as part of the importance of changing lifestyle. In other words, to make a bridge between his powerful feelings and her own agenda.*
Nurse	Yes, right, something to stay fit for. Yes.	
David	But other than that, you know, family stuff is good.	*He accepts the move back to agenda setting.*
Nurse	Food, we talked about.	*Continues completing chart.*
David	Yes.	
Nurse	Smoking. Smoking is the number one from our point of view, but it's not always the one that people want to start with.	*Offers information on the importance of smoking but conveys that it is up to him to decide where to start.*
David	Smoking is more important than the food and that?	*Asking for information.*
Nurse	It's the biggest single thing you can do to benefit your health.	*Gives information clearly but briefly.*
David	Right. [Sighs]	
Nurse	But it's not, not everybody finds that the easiest one to start with.	*Responds to his nonverbal signs of resistance.*
David	So…	
Nurse	So, tell me where you'd like to start.	*This is a critical question. She keeps focus on behavior change but gives him control about the specific agenda.*
David	Them two are connected. Stress and smoking.	*Offers information about how smoking fits into his life and his priorities.*
Nurse	Are they for you? You smoke when you're stressed?	*Follows and asks for elaboration.*
David	I think so yes. I smoke all the time but, I think I would be even more stressed if I tried to stop smoking, you know what I mean.	
Nurse	Right, OK. Leave that for now. Exercise is another one. How active are you physically?	*Recognizes resistance and switches to another option on the agenda-setting chart.*

David	Well, I've got quite a physical job. But that's about it. I don't really have much time to do anything else. I'm not really the sort of person that goes down the gym. I have always thought that I was quite healthy anyway. Not healthy obviously, smoking's not healthy, but quite fit. Just sort of naturally, but obviously I was wrong, you know what I mean?	
Nurse	Before you were ill, how would you have been if you were kind of running up a flight of stairs or running to catch a train?	*Follows his initiative in assessing how much fitness is an issue for him.*
David	Probably a bit below average I think. I would get out of breath I guess. Yes. I just, I used to play football and that when I was younger, but I don't now.	
Nurse	It's all kind of gone on the back burner a bit.	*Reflection.*
David	Yes, I don't do anything now. But as I say, my job is quite physical. You know, doing people's lofts out, a lot of stairs getting into the loft or climbing the ladders and that, it's quite a physical job sometimes.	
Nurse	That sounds like, if you are getting out of breath still, it might be that it builds up your strength but not so much your stamina.	
David	Could be, yes.	
Nurse	Those would be the main things. We talked about alcohol. Alcohol is less of a risk factor for heart disease. It is actually a risk factor for other things.	*Avoiding a premature focus on the exercise issue, moves back to agenda-setting chart and exchanging information.*
David	Right.	
Nurse	So, I am not saying it's a kind of good thing to do too much.	
David	You are not suggesting I have more alcohol and…	
Nurse	Absolutely not. But it's kind of, just in terms of heart disease which we are talking about today, it's a lesser factor.	*Keeps focus on the cardiac issues.*
David	So we won't worry about that one for now?	
Nurse	What do you think if you look at all those and you put any more in that you want to put in, where would you think would be somewhere, with the life that you have got, where would be somewhere you could start to kind of look after yourself a little bit more. Keep yourself well?	*She returns to the core question about where would he like to start making changes.*

David	I guess food, I mean food's something I could... looking at... what I normally do is, if I am working which I am pretty much, 6 sometimes 7 days a week, but generally 6 days a week. I don't have a lunch break as such, you know. I just get one of the lads to run out to get me a burger or something. There's a burger place just opposite where our office is, so that's the easiest thing, get a burger or something like that. Just easy, I can eat it when I am working. Get some chips with it in there. That's pretty much what I do.	*He is more motivated to work on his food than anything else (or at least less reluctant!)*
Nurse	Right, so that's tangled up with stress as well. These are all having a knock on effect on each other aren't they? You're stressed at work so you don't eat well.	*Good example of how items on the agenda are often interrelated.*
David	Well it's all connected isn't it? I am at work, I am getting stressed out, so busy, someone runs out, gets me a burger. Quickly eat the burger while I am working.	*He expresses concern rather than the nurse.*
Nurse	Yes.	
David	It's just easy; don't have to worry about it. It's just there, on a plate for you, as it were.	
Nurse	It is literally, yes! So, you picked that one as being one you might be able to do something about. What...	*About to inquire into importance and confidence.*
David	I am just thinking, I don't want to give up smoking.	*Interrupts with resistance.*
Nurse	Right, OK, fair enough. That feels like too hard at the moment.	*Rolls with the resistance with a reflection without dismissing it as a topic for another time.*
David	I just think it will get me even more stressed now. The whole thing has set me back you know. It's got me thinking about you know. Having a heart attack and that. That has stressed me out even more. And when I am stressed out, I have a smoke, because it helps me relax you know. I know it's ridiculous but everyone says it, it's bad for you and I know it's bad for you. But it does, it helps me relax at the minute. Maybe that's more for one I can think about later on.	

Nurse	Right, put that on the back burner for now and come back to that one.	
David	Yes, maybe.	
Nurse	The food...	*Still looking to see if there is a topic he is ready to discuss.*
David	I wish there was like a magic pill that I could take it all away, you know what I mean.	*Resistance emerging again; he seems overwhelmed by the thought of so much change.*
Nurse	I know. Yes.	*Rolls with the resistance.*
David	All these things like a bit...	
Nurse	It's kind of hard, yes. If you could just take a pill every day and it would sort it all out, it would be an easy option for you. Yes.	
David	Do you think they're going to invent one then? [Laughs]	*Acknowledges, via joking, that he knows he's got to look at the lifestyle issues.*
Nurse	They might do eventually but I suspect not. Meanwhile, this is the stuff that needs looking at. If you were thinking about eating differently to benefit your heart, would there be any other benefits in eating differently for you? Or in any of these? Can you see any kind of... well thinking "It's for my heart but, I would also get something else out of it"?	*Loses congruence briefly, trying to keep to the agenda. Begins exploration of importance of eating differently as he seems to have chosen this as the place to start.*
David	Well, if I tried to give myself like a proper you know, lunch break you know, just said "Right this is my lunch break, I am having my lunch. Phone off the hook, I am not available. I am going to have half an hour. Not going to think about work." I say that sitting here though but, you know what I mean. It's easy enough to say it here. But maybe that could be part of, we could work toward that.	*Sets himself a target; stop work for half an hour and have a healthy lunch.*
Nurse	And what would you eat in that break? What would be feasible for you? You obviously need a lot of energy with the job, so you are not going to be starving yourself. Good healthy stuff. What do you know about the sorts of foods that are good for your heart?	*Exchanging information about healthy eating with a view to coming up with strategies for meeting his target.*

David	Fruit and stuff I am guessing. Is it?	*Seeking information.*
Nurse	Fruit and veg.	
David	Fruit and veg.	*Resistance waiting in the wings here.*
		Providing information.
Nurse	Anything that's not too fatty. The biggest enemy is things very greasy, things like you say, burgers, anything that's been fried or with loads of butter on.	
David	All the stuff I've been eating for the last 30 years.	
Nurse	And that's a very common thing in your line of business. It's classic; lots of calories and grab it quick.	*Trying to convey a nonjudgmental approach by talking about his eating habits as normal or commonplace.*
David	And I guess what I should be doing is make — bring stuff from home isn't it? Like making something in the mornings.	*Now he's got the information about healthy eating, he starts to explore strategies.*
Nurse	Well, that would save you the time thing, because it sounds like you don't want to go walking round trying to find a café somewhere.	*Supports his ideas.*
David	So, I don't know. I am saying bring a salad and that, thinking — can't just have a salad for lunch can you? Well I can't.	*Resistance emerges again once he thinks about the reality of what he's suggesting.*
Nurse	What about sandwiches? Is there any sort of sandwich that you could eat?	*Shifts to other options rather than engaging in a debate about salad which might increase resistance.*
David	Sandwiches are better for you, like?	*Seeking information again.*
Nurse	Depends what you put in them.	
David	Can't put a burger in it? [Laughs]	
Nurse	Absolutely not. Burger butties, chip butties!	*Responds to request for information.*
David	Can I have cheese, is cheese all right?	*Still pursuing and receptive to information.*
Nurse	Some cheeses are much lower fat than others.	*Responds with further information.*
David	Right, low-fat cheese.	
Nurse	So, things like…	
David	That's what my missus has.	*He is considering possibilities. It seems it is important to him to change and he's struggling to see how to make it a reality. It is not so much resistance as a genuine vocalization of his difficulty imagining building healthy eating into his life.*

Nurse	Low-fat cheese?	
David	Well, she has them spreads. I'm not really into those spread things. You know what I mean.	*Back come the objections. He cannot picture himself doing what is being asked of him.*
Nurse	Sounds as if you, your wife is quite conscious about low-fat food then, is she, for herself?	*Reflection, drawing his attention to his wife as a potential source of information and support. Possibility of this building confidence.*
David	Yes, she looks after herself. Yes.	
Nurse	So, she knows all, she would be able to help you.	
David	She probably would, yes.	
Nurse	About thinking about all of this.	
David	Probably be blooming amazed. She would say, "What are you doing?"	
Nurse	But she would be a support to you in terms of having the knowledge to…	*Building confidence by exploring a source of support.*
David	Yes, she is as worried as I am about this whole thing happening. I mean, yes. I mean, I could probably ask her to, you know, help me out. Sandwiches then is it?	*Sees the possibility but is reluctant to commit.*
Nurse	Well let's have a think, that's one option. Let's think of some more options for what you can eat. Does anybody else you work with tend to take their own?	*In the face of resistance, doesn't push it.*
David	No, I am working with… most of the lads I work with, you know, are young lads, so, yes. You know, haven't got a care in the world have they? When I was 17, 18 I didn't give a monkey's what I ate you know what I mean? Whatever you want — chocolate, packet of crisps, chips to keep you going. Some of them don't even have lunch you know what I mean, just smoke their way through lunch. All part of it, all part of the environment in which I am working. Because the thing about smoking, you know for what I do, smoking is, you know, a 5-min break.	*Gives the nurse valuable information about his life and the context in which he will be trying to make these changes.*

Nurse	Yes.	
David	You need that 5-min break throughout the day.	*His objection to changing what he eats is now showing in the form of switching the conversation to talking about smoking! Lighthearted reflection acknowledging that a lot is being asked of him.*
Nurse	Yes, so your breaks are all associated with the things that aren't very good for your heart!	
David	They seem to be don't they. There's no hope for me. [Laughs]	
Nurse	Stop for a smoke, stop for a burger or go to the pub yes. Well sandwiches are a good option because bread is quite filling. If you can think of low-fat things, if your wife can help you think of low-fat things. And stick some salady things in. Fruit is really good, I don't know how much of a fruit eater you are.	*Directs the conversation back to the agenda with a summary of options they've considered so far. Then moves to exchanging information about more options.*
David	Yes, fruit is all right, yes.	
Nurse	You can eat tons of that. You don't have to just have an apple. You can…	
David	Keep scoffing it can you?	
Nurse	Yes, absolutely.	
David	Right… get a bit of fruit inside me.	
Nurse	All right, so it looks as if for the moment…	*Thinks, mistakenly, that he has accepted her suggestions and an agreement has been reached!*
David	It's a big change that, isn't it? Going from burgers to sandwiches and that.	*No, he really hasn't come to terms with this yet and is resisting being nudged forward into a plan.*
Nurse	Well it is, yes. Does that feel almost too much to do?	*Technically a closed question but with the intention of restoring congruence.*
David	No, I suppose it's important isn't it. I don't want to end up where I ended up a few weeks ago, do I? The last thing I want. I don't want my kids coming in, seeing me laying out in a hospital. Looking like a, I don't know. It must have scared them.	*Congruence restored, resistance settles down again and David reminds himself why they are having this conversation.*

Nurse	Must have scared them.	*Reflection.*
David	It scared me, I am telling you. I don't mind admitting it did. I was terrified.	*This can be seen as change talk. He is giving himself good reason to make the behavior change.*
Nurse	OK, so we've agreed that the food is the best place to start. Particularly lunches. Can I ask you some questions to get a feel of it? How important... if I asked you how important it was for you to start to eat differently, since you had the heart attack, on a scale of 1–10. 1 is it's not important at all and 10 is it's really important, where would you put it at the moment?	*Faced with such mixed messages from him about his willingness to change, tries a scaling question to clarify.*
David	Well, if it's going to make a difference you know. Umm, about 9 or 10. It's pretty important isn't it?	*The scaling has moved him away from resistance again.*
Nurse	And it's as high as that because of your fear that you talked about.	*Reflection of previous change talk.*
David	Yes.	
Nurse	How it's really shaken you up.	*Further reflection.*
David	If I can change what I'm eating at lunch time and that will, you know, cut down the chances of this happening to me again...then it's a 10.	
Nurse	It's a 10. So, if you are absolutely sure it will make a difference, yes. OK, that's something we would be able to measure, the difference, because we can measure what level of things are in your blood.	*Reflection and information exchange.*
David	Oh right.	
Nurse	So we can actually check your cholesterol levels, and give you some feedback as to whether...	*Recognizes that he needs evidence that he is achieving his goal, i.e., reducing the risk of another heart attack.*
David	Whether it's actually doing anything?	
Nurse	If it's working, yes. And if I was going to ask another similar question, 1–10 question but say this time how confident are you that you could do it? How do you feel? 1 is I can't do it and 10 is yes, if I make my mind up. If you made your mind up and were determined, do you think you could do it? Where would you...	

David	About 5.	
Nurse	A 50:50 chance.	*Reflection.*
David	Yes it's like, I know what I should be doing. It's like smoking. I know I shouldn't be smoking but I still do it. It's like I know what I should be doing. I know I should be changing what I am eating. So that's the 5 bit. It's the actually sitting in the office, with phones going and people coming in and problems mounting up and, it's…	*Elaborates.*
Nurse	So, it sounds like you, it might not be that much of a priority. Hard to keep it a priority when you are in work, when you are busy.	*Reflection. Importance and confidence somewhat intertwined at this point.*
David	That's it.	
Nurse	It's a priority now because you are sitting in a health setting…	
David	That's it.	
Nurse	…talking about your heart.	*Following, so as to understand his position better.*
David	Exactly yes. And it was only a few weeks ago, wasn't it. But in 4–5 months time. You know, a heart attack could seem a thing of the past.	
Nurse	Yes and that does happen for a lot of people.	
David	It might be that I can do it for, you know, 2 weeks, 3 weeks. Another thing you have got to bear in mind is I am going to get some right stick from the lads. You know, if I start eating fruit. That sounds funny doesn't it, but…	*As he pictures himself sitting in the office with an apple he discovers another obstacle; the risk of being ridiculed.*
Nurse	Yes, well that's a concern, but on the other hand, when you say 50:50, that's half of you thinks you can do it.	*Moves back to "Why so high?" to elicit the change talk side of the inner conflict.*
David	Yes, that's true.	
Nurse	So it's kind of…	
David	Because it's that half I need to be…	
Nurse	Yes, what's that half about? What's the bit of you, the bit that says it's important and you want to do it?	*Goes back to importance.*

David	Yes, and the bit about being scared. You know. Like I said before I don't, I don't want to end up, I don't want to be sitting here again in 2 years time having the same conversation. You know what I mean. I don't want that.	*Confirms importance.*
Nurse	No.	
David	Because if I am, no offense to you, but if I am, it means I have had another heart attack.	
Nurse	Absolutely yes, we like it when we don't see people again.	
David	Yes.	
Nurse	Yes. So confidence in terms of it's important to you. What about in terms of it actually being possible to get your sarnies (sandwiches) together and go to work, and have a proper break. How possible does that feel?	*Having confirmed importance, moves back to confidence.*
David	Well getting the sarnies done is no problem cause you know my, my wife, we do it anyway. She has sandwiches, the kids have sandwiches for school. So it's just like…	
Nurse	There's a system there.	*Reflection.*
David	It's all set up. You know what I mean, it's not a problem. It's like, you know, I just haven't bothered before. So, actually at work I think that's going to be the biggest issue. You know, actually going, I am having half an hour, eating my sandwiches…	
Nurse	Right, so it's actually taking the time out. The sarnies, presumably once they are there, it's easier than sending for a burger.	
David	Yes if they are there…	
Nurse	It's not that, kind of, not that, that's an issue. You will eat them, it's whether you actually take a break.	
David	The trouble is, what I might do is I might eat them about 11 and then still have a burger. [Laughs]	
Nurse	So you need to take plenty.	
David	Yes.	
Nurse	Right. And you are not overweight so we are not worried about the quantity that you are eating.	*Providing information.*
David	No, I don't think I'm overweight.	

Nurse	If you eat more healthy food, that's not an issue, your weight, so that's not something you have to worry about.	*Providing information.*
David	OK.	
Nurse	OK, so it's really important for you to do it.	*Begins to summarize.*
David	Yes, definitely.	
Nurse	It's just the kind of day-to-day trying it out, see how it goes.	
David	Yes, I guess that's all I can do and I have got to give it a go.	
Nurse	Yes.	
David	There is no point me sitting here and saying "Oh yes, it's very straightforward for me." There is no point in me telling you that is there, because that's not true. I actually think it's going to be quite hard.	
Nurse	Yes.	
David	It might sound stupid to…	
Nurse	Well, breaking habits is hard, it's always hard.	*Seeking to encourage without giving unrealistic assurances.*
David	That's what it is, isn't it. It's like a habit. That's what it feels like.	
Nurse	Always hard. Yes, as I say, if we keep in touch we can, like when things, next time, to find out what's difficult. You might find, some people find that some things they thought would be really difficult are quite easy and some things that they thought would be easy are quite difficult. We can kind of see how it's going and talk it through a bit.	
David	OK, good.	
Nurse	All right.	
David	Thank you.	

REFERENCE

Gilligan, T., Mason, P., 2006. Engaging Motivation DVD. Pip Mason Consultancy Ltd., Birmingham.

Discussion sheet Ms Rees

13

CHAPTER OUTLINE

Ms Rees's asthma is poorly controlled. In the asthma clinic she is asked about her smoking.
Sheet to be used alongside watching the video example in http://evolve.elsevier.com/Mason/healthbehavior/. It can either provide a structure for private study or for team development.

WHAT DOES THIS CONSULTATION ILLUSTRATE?

This is an example of the whole process of the consultation, from *establishing rapport* through to *closing*, incorporating, along the way, *exchanging information* and *rolling with resistance*. When watching, you might find it helpful to have the diagram on the *overview of the consultation* (see p. 7) in front of you.

CONSIDER THE FOLLOWING

How does the practitioner establish rapport and raise the issue?
She raises the issue of smoking after first discussing inhaler use. Would it have made a difference if it had been the other way around? Why? How?
The practitioner uses scaling questions to explore importance, confidence, and readiness. She asked "*What puts you just past the halfway mark*?" Instead she could have asked "*Why are you not any higher than that?*" What would have been different if she had phrased it like that?
The practitioner asks Ms Rees whether there are any reasons apart from health for giving up smoking. She could, instead, have told her the reasons or given a leaflet on the topic. What difference does it make?
How does the practitioner roll with the patient's resistance?

What do you think about the way the practitioner gave the information about smoking cessation services? Could she/should she have given it a harder sell? How do you feel about the way the consultation ended?

Taken with permission from Mason, P., Butler, C.H., 2011. Ready, Willing and Able Learning Pack. Pip Mason Consultancy Ltd., Birmingham.

Appendices: patient worksheets

Throughout the text, we have suggested visual aids to use when talking with patients. In the text, we illustrated these possibilities. On the following pages, we provide larger scale master copies of these worksheets that you can photocopy to use in your consultations. To get best value from them, do not use them before reading the relevant chapter for each.

These are also all available on the website (http://evolve.elsevier.com/Mason/healthbehavior/) for you to download and print.

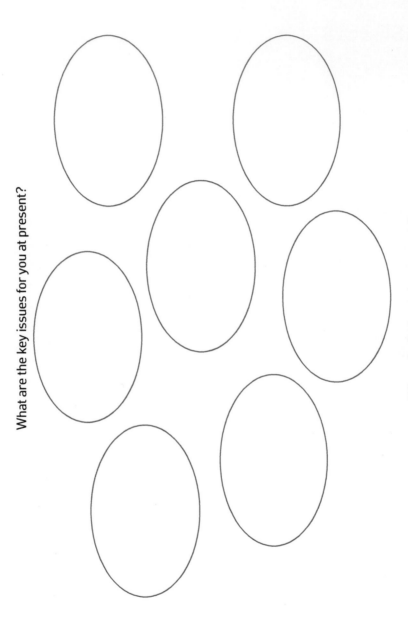

What are the key issues for you at present?

Where is the best place to start?

FIGURE 1

Agenda-setting chart.

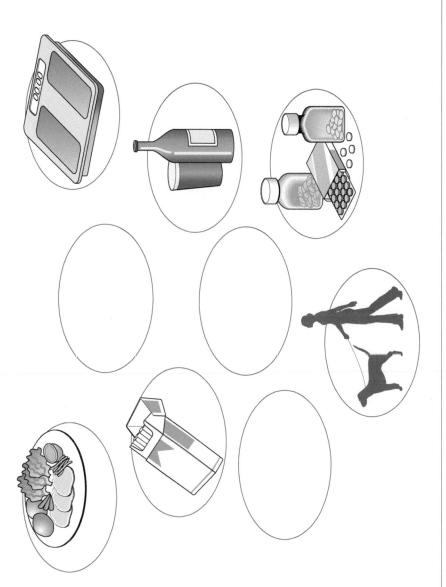

FIGURE 2

Proforma agenda setting chart.

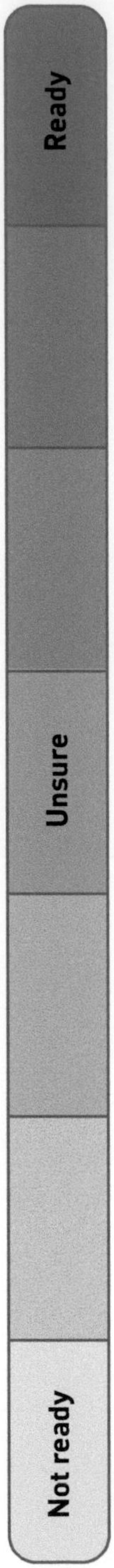

FIGURE 3

Readiness rule.

Unimportant ———————————————— **Top priority**

How important is it to you to change?
Put a cross on the line to represent how you feel

I couldn't do it ———————————————— **It would be easy**

How confident are you that you could
change if you chose to?
Put a cross on the line to represent how you feel

FIGURE 4

Importance and confidence continuum.

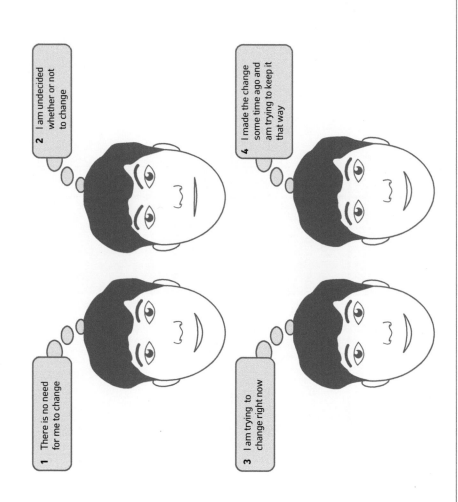

FIGURE 5

Little faces chart.

No change	Change
Costs	Costs
Benefits	Benefits

FIGURE 6
Balance sheet.

Goal (general)	**Strategies** (specific)	**Targets** (very specific)

FIGURE 7

Goals, strategies, and targets chart.

Index